"Intense, controversial, loud and clear . . .
A chronicle of tenacity and courage."
—*Virginian Pilot*

The great granddaughter of slaves and the impoverished child of Arkansas sharecroppers, Joycelyn Elders grew up in a three-room shack with no electricity or plumbing. Until she entered college, she had never seen a doctor, let alone dreamed of becoming one. Yet after enrolling in medical school in 1956 as the only black woman in her class, she went on to become one of the most prominent pediatric endocrinologists in the United States, and the first woman to assume the role of U.S. Surgeon General. Told in Elders's powerful, plainspoken voice, the story of her pioneering journey to the highest medical position in the country dramatizes the themes that have informed her life: the power of a loving family, education, and the resources of the human spirit. In this profoundly uplifting and unforgettable memoir, Dr. Elders reveals how she found the courage to remain true to herself and her beliefs, even in the face of personal tragedy and fierce political opposition. Bracingly candid and genuine, JOYCELYN ELDERS, M.D., will take its place as a classic account of the triumphant rise of a role model and a truly inspirational American woman.

"May make readers wish that her voice was still audible in the Surgeon General's office and not merely in the pages of this inspiring memoir."
—*People*

"Charming . . . the former Surgeon General delivers a folksy life story . . . Though she frequently and proudly refers to her outspoken nature, she maintains on the printed page an appealing humility."
—*The New York Times Book Review*

JOYCELYN ELDERS, M.D.

FROM
SHARECROPPER'S
DAUGHTER TO
SURGEON GENERAL
OF THE
UNITED STATES
OF AMERICA

DR. JOYCELYN ELDERS

AND

DAVID CHANOFF

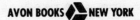
AVON BOOKS ◆ NEW YORK

AVON BOOKS
A division of
The Hearst Corporation
1350 Avenue of the Americas
New York, New York 10019

Published in hardcover by William Morrow and Company, Inc.; for information address Permissions Department, William Morrow and Company, Inc., 1350 Avenue of the Americas, New York, New York 10019.

The William Morrow edition contains the following Library of Congress Cataloging in Publication Data:

Elders, M. Joycelyn.
   Joycelyn Elders, M. D. : from sharecropper's daughter to surgeon general of the United States of America / Joycelyn Elders and David Chanoff.—1st ed.
     p.   cm.
1. Elders, M. Joycelyn. 2. Health officers—United Sates—Biography. 3. Women physicians—Arkansas—Biography. 4. Afro-American physicians—Arkansas—Biography. I. Chanoff, David. II. Title.
R154.E48A3   1996
610'.92—dc20   96-9036
[B]   CIP

First Avon Books Trade Printing: October 1997

AVON TRADEMARK REG. U.S. PAT. OFF. AND IN OTHER COUNTRIES, MARCA REGISTRADA, HECHO EN U.S.A.

Printed in the U.S.A.

OPM 10 9 8 7 6 5 4 3 2 1

This book is dedicated to my mother, Haller Jones (1912–1995), for four gifts of wisdom she gave to me that served me well throughout my life and especially during the most difficult and trying times.

If you want to get out of the fields, get something in your head.

Recognize the truth and speak out against wrongdoing.

Don't use up your future trying to recapture the past.

Do your best; that's good enough.

Acknowledgments

Many people whose lives have intersected with mine over the years shared their memories with David Chanoff and me as we were writing. Among my family we especially want to thank my husband, Oliver; my brother Chester Jones; my aunt Joella Sowell; my uncles Reva and Gus Jones; and my brother Phillip Jones. Others to whom we owe a large debt for filling out my own recollection of events with their often broader and more detailed memories are Tom Butler, Dr. Ed Hughes, Dr. Edith Irby Jones, Barbara Kilgore, Jennifer Hui, Dr. Lee Lee Doyle, Nancy Kirsch, Bill Hamilton, George Harper, Senator Jay Bradford, Louise Dennis, Joyce Gibson, Willie Mitchum, Ernie Dumas, Bob McCord, and Mary Ann Chaffee.

Our thanks go as well to Geleve Grice, the Reverend Dorothy Asare, Professor Willard Gatewood of the University of Arkansas, Dr. John Parascandola of the United States Commissioned Corps, and Drs. Thoru Pederson and John McCracken of the Worcester Foundation for Biomedical Research for help in clarifying some of the historical and technical background that found its way into the book. We also wish to express our sincere gratitude to the Sisters' Fund for its generous support of this project.

Rob Stewart and Molly Chanoff were wonderfully efficient transcribers. Olli Chanoff provided research assistance. Thanks to them for having made our work go faster and more easily than it otherwise would have. Ellen Simmons and Avi Eden read the manuscript and gave us thoughtful and unsparing editorial advice, one of friendship's more difficult burdens.

Finally, we want to thank our agent, Owen Laster, for his support and enthusiasm along the way. At William Morrow, Tracy Quinn handled all the often hectic details with skill and exemplary calm. Claire Wachtel, our editor, has the sharp eye and light touch every writer prays for but few have the good luck ever to experience.

Contents

Introduction

During the Senate debate over my confirmation as surgeon general in August 1993 some strange things happened. At one point, after Republican senators had been attacking me for a while, Carol Moseley-Braun, the junior Democrat from Illinois, got the floor. She was mad. She said the debate had turned into lies and character assassination. She said it had become an inquisition and that she didn't know who exactly was vying for the Torquemada Award, but that somebody ought to get it.

When she said that, Don Nickles from Oklahoma stood up and accused her of violating Rule 19, which is the rule against senators slandering other senators. Moseley-Braun hadn't mentioned any names, but Nickles was one of the main ones doing the attacking right then, along with Trent Lott of Mississippi. So Nickles got up and said, "Rule Nineteen." When Ted Kennedy heard that, he called out, "Regular order," meaning that the acting chairman should tell Nickles he was out of order and give the floor back to Moseley-Braun. Then John McCain, the Republican from Arizona, jumped up from where he was sitting on the other side of the aisle, and *he* started yelling, "Regular order!" meaning the chairman should tell Kennedy to sit down and they should get back to Nickles.

I wasn't in the Senate chamber at the time so I didn't see this myself, though it's printed in the *Congressional Record*. According to a friend of mine who was in the gallery, McCain went red in the face and stormed across the way toward Kennedy so angry it looked like he might hit him. When he got there, he said what sounded like "Why don't you shut up, you bully? You're always bossing everybody around," or words to that effect. And Kennedy said, "Why don't *you* shut up?" My friend was wondering what would happen if McCain actually punched Kennedy. Would they somehow be able to turn off the C-Span cameras? Meanwhile the chairman was calling for order and saying, "All senators will suspend!," which meant they had to stop what they were doing and get back to being senators. After that everybody backed off some, but their hackles were still up. Then Phil Gramm from Texas gave a speech that cooled everyone down a little, which gives you an idea how hot they were.

John McCain opposed my confirmation, and Ted Kennedy was fighting hard for me, but they were probably both surprised to find themselves face-to-face like that. McCain is known to get emotional, but he is basically a courteous and friendly man, as I knew from the times I had testified before him earlier. And though conservatives may not like Kennedy's positions, I think everyone sees him as an especially collegial senator. So they might not have recognized themselves in that confrontation.

In a lot of the controversy over my nomination I could scarcely recognize myself. What people might have thought who didn't know me but only read the newspapers I can't even begin to imagine. I have been a churchgoing, believing Christian all my life, but Pat Buchanan was writing that I was a leader of "post-Christian paganism." I grew up in a sharecropper's shack in southwestern Arkansas during segregation, but Alan Keyes had me down as someone who believed that "the lives of oppressed people are worthless" and that people who might "be born into poverty and suffering aren't worth saving." I had spent a large part of my professional life as a pediatrician and medical scientist working to save newborn babies and trying to give children with congenital defects full and healthy lives. But Senator

Nickles was accusing me of wanting to kill off babies with defects before they were born. Maybe I would even consider it a good idea, he told the Senate, to give babies a month or two after they were born to find out if they had a real problem and then kill them.

I knew what Everett Koop had gone through in his confirmation. I had talked to him and read his book. So I was prepared for a rough time. Plus I had just spent six years arguing health issues in the Arkansas legislature, where they believe that politics is a body contact sport. But a Senate confirmation hearing just isn't something you can train for. One veteran of these things told me it's rare to have a nominee who's so unqualified that that's what the debate is actually about. In any nomination of a person, personalities are the issue. It's not like considering a missile treaty, for instance, where there are objective criteria you can use. What it comes down to is who likes the nominee, who doesn't, and why.

I don't think anybody truly believed I wasn't qualified to be surgeon general, even though Senator John Danforth of Missouri did say I was "startlingly unqualified" and Dan Coats of Indiana seemed to have a hard time believing I was actually a doctor; at one point he asked about what nursing duties I had performed. I think those and some similar things Jesse Helms said were aberrations. On the other hand, there were issues my nomination raised that people felt very strongly about, personal issues with major policy ramifications. Sex education and teenage pregnancy, for example, abortion and AIDS and condoms in schools. Even Christian morality.

In my six years as director of Arkansas's health department, I had become a lightning rod on these issues. That was ironic in a way, because for the quarter century before that as a professor of pediatric endocrinology what I mainly saw was the inside of my laboratory, my classroom, and my clinic. In that whole time I probably hadn't ever spent more than five minutes at a stretch thinking about public health. The biggest controversy I ever got into might have been over whether we could get some day care started at the medical school. But once I moved over to the health department I landed in the middle of a national debate on values that looked more like a war than an argument.

While that debate had different components, near its heart was how people think about sex: how to teach children about it, what sexual responsibility means, and the consequences of unmarried and unprotected sexual activity for public health. Swirling around in this mix were issues like AIDS, abortion, homosexuality, and sexual abuse, which meant there was never any lack of people who were seriously disturbed about something.

The fact that I was the one at the center of these sex wars was ironic in another way too. When I was growing up in Schaal, Arkansas, sex was so secret that no adult ever mentioned it, period. Somewhere in the United States there might have been a child more ignorant about sex than I was, but you'd have been hard pressed to find her. By contrast, later on, when I became a doctor, part of my job was to treat all the really severe problems of sexual development in Arkansas, from babies born with ambiguous genitalia to children who never went into puberty. At one time I had more experience talking to parents and children about sex than any doctor in the state and probably as much as anyone in the country. In those days there weren't more than a handful of specialists who knew much about these things.

Maybe it was because of my background that I never stopped being exasperated by all the commotion over condoms and sex education. I knew firsthand what it is like to be ignorant, and I also knew how vital it is to be informed. When I was health director, we were seeing frightening increases in AIDS cases and an epidemic of pregnancy among unmarried teenagers that was eating at the country's social fabric. But hysteria about sex was disabling our primary means of prevention, which is of course just as true today. No health professional can really tolerate that. My predecessor as surgeon general, Antonia Novello, couldn't any more than Koop or I could, although we each had our own ways of trying to contend with it.

Maybe even worse was that by focusing attention on subjects

like abortion and sex education, the loud right-wing groups were distorting and politicizing health issues generally. What I hated as much as anything about my confirmation debate was that most of the other side was so preoccupied with sex issues that they didn't care in the slightest what I might have actually done for public health in Arkansas, most of which had nothing to do with sexuality.

While I was director there, we had raised our childhood immunization rate from 34 to 60 percent—96 percent for first graders. Our early-childhood health screening was twelve times what it had been. We set up sickle-cell anemia screening and a comprehensive women's health program. Our prenatal care rate went way up, as did the numbers of qualifying women getting food supplements for their children. We built a major in-home health service to care for our frail and elderly, and we made a lot of headway in attracting doctors to rural areas that didn't have any. We established home hospice care and got the churches involved in that. We built twenty-eight new public health clinics, renovated fourteen more, and opened twenty-four clinics in schools. I was proud of what we had accomplished. I thought the health department had improved the lives of a lot of Arkansans. But none of that made a whit of difference to people who were fixated on abortion and couldn't bear the thought of sex education.

Of course I have to admit I didn't make it easy for them. I had been up on the barricades a long time, and when I thought strong language was needed, I didn't shy from it. I wasn't a stealth candidate for surgeon general. A lot of what I had said was public record, and a few of my comments had really lodged in some throats. During the confirmation debate those were the ones that got repeated over and over again, most often out of context and twisted.

In one speech I had said that we've taught teenagers what to do in the front seat of cars, now we have to teach them what to do in the back, meaning that if we were instructing them on traffic safety, we surely ought to be teaching them how to protect themselves from AIDS and other sexually transmitted diseases

(STDs) and pregnancy. I had said that girls going out on prom dates should carry condoms in their purses, meaning that if there was any chance they weren't going to be abstinent, they should be ready with contraception. Senators Trent Lott and Don Nickles and a couple of others believed comments like those showed I was advocating immorality. They seemed to think, like Pat Buchanan did, that I saw teenagers mainly as "rutting animals whom we expect to do a good deal of fornicating."

Worse, I had taken to calling the extremist right-to-life groups "very religious non-Christians," and more than once I had said they should "get over their love affair with the fetus." The first time Senator Coats brought those up to me, I told him that in Arkansas the groups I was talking about "fight against health education, they fight against welfare, they fight against Medicaid. They always want to have the children born, but they don't want to support them after they're here. That's an affair," I told him. "That's a short-term commitment, whereas with children that's forever. In my state," I said, "I have not seen these people out working for programs to help poor children and mothers. If we had a society where everybody was provided health care, a decent place to live, and adequate education, then, Senator, we would be taking care of people. But in my state I don't see these kinds of commitments." That was pretty much the tone of the whole debate. It was tense and confrontational.

My opponents said they were outraged by the language I used. They were offended. Even some of my supporters thought I might do well to tone it down. Senator Nancy Kassebaum of Kansas, who was a voice in my corner, said maybe I needed to work on my bedside manner, and David Pryor, one of Arkansas's two wonderful senators, mentioned that I had a number of diplomas but I didn't have one from the school of diplomacy. But others said that in their opinion, using plain, unvarnished English was a virtue, and they wished more government people would do it. My favorite was Barbara Boxer, who said she wasn't offended by my language. What she was offended by was that the infant mortality rate in the United States was higher than in nineteen other countries and that the black infant mortality rate was higher than in thirty-one other countries, including Cuba and Bulgaria. She was offended that we ranked thirty-first in low-birth-weight babies and seventeenth in polio immunization and that the American preschool death rate was twentieth in the world. With that kind of record, she didn't have time to be offended by someone's language.

———

Bill Clinton's military adviser Admiral William Crowe said once that in all his many years of testifying in Congress he could maybe recall one person whose mind he might have changed on something, but he wasn't sure. For all the debate over my nomination, no one I can think of changed sides. Nobody won any converts by being more logical and cogent than somebody else.

But as another Washington person told me, what happens in the Senate may not be an elegant intellectual argument, but it is extremely sophisticated political choreography. If a Fritz Hollings or John Glenn won't get up and speak for you, that could mean you don't have the conservative Democrats. Maybe there's a weakness, and the other side can build some kind of negative momentum that will tip things against you.

Well, we did get Fritz Hollings and John Glenn, plus Republicans like Mark Hatfield and Alan Simpson and David Durenberger. And every Republican we got was a shot below the waterline. Ted Kennedy, who shepherded my confirmation, was a master at these things. If you ever need an advocate on the floor of the Senate, you can't get anyone better. He's a fighter. When all the talk finally stopped, the vote was 65 to 34 with 12 Republicans voting yea.

Afterward President Clinton told me he thought it was wonderful we had won. I said, "Mr. President, I'm glad you thought that what happened was wonderful because I sure didn't."

"You know," I told my husband, Oliver, "I went in there feeling like prime steak, and I came out feeling like poor-grade hamburger."

At one point in the debate Ted Kennedy had said they were

7

going to be voting on the real Joycelyn Elders, not some unrecognizable straw woman. But when it was over, I wasn't positive people knew who I was much better than they had when it started. After only fifteen months as surgeon general, I'm not sure they ever really did get to find out.

Chapter 1

Schaal

❧

The town of Schaal, Arkansas, where I was born on August 13, 1933, has a population of ninety-eight, ninety-nine when I'm home. Schaal is too small for most maps, especially since the Williams brothers' general store burned down and the post office moved to Mineral Springs. The only other enterprises in town were the cotton gin and a little ground hog sawmill, and they too are long gone.

To get to Schaal, you take the interstate west out of Little Rock. The moment you branch off onto Route 24, you're deep in the country. The white oak and pine woods look just like they did in my childhood. So do the fenced pastures with their little knots of cattle. When the more prosperous farms near the interstate give out, you begin to see wooden shacks and churches—tiny white buildings scattered along the highway at quicker intervals than you might expect. The churches aren't much bigger than the houses. The only real difference is there's a steeple on top and a name over the door: Sweet Home Baptist, Calvary Methodist, AME Zion, Church of Christ, Assembly of God, Church of God in Christ.

Heading toward Nashville and Mineral Springs, you feel like you're going back to an earlier time. On Sundays the churches are full. If you turn off the air conditioning in your car and open the windows, you can hear snatches of singing as you drive by. All along Route 24 the air is humming with old hymns.

Nashville, not the big one in Tennessee, but the little one near Schaal, is where the black kids from the farms used to go on special occasions when I was young. You saved your pennies and Edmund Turner came around in his battered bus and picked you up, the same bus he used to take children to school and workers out to migrant labor jobs picking cotton in Arizona or tomatoes in Ohio. In Nashville we'd walk around staring in the store windows and maybe see a movie at the Rialto—from up in the balcony in those days of segregation. That was a once- or twice-a-year thing. That was our idea of a good time, strolling the sidewalks, getting a Popsicle or a soda, checking out every-body else, even if half of them were your cousins to one degree or another. You saved up hard for that.

Drive down the winding dirt road toward Schaal, and you are about as far from Washington, D.C., as you can get. If you're from here and old enough like I am to remember before tractors and electrification, the surprise is how little it's changed. It takes no trouble at all to picture in your imagination large families working in the fields, children and adults together, everyone trooping back home at sundown to bathe in the round tin tubs that were set out on the back porch all day so the water could catch the heat of the sun. That's what I did from the time I could walk in the furrows until the day I left home for college when I was sixteen. I'd throw my sweated-through, dirt-caked field dress in the washpot for boiling and blueing; then I climbed into a tub and scrubbed hard. The idea wasn't just to get clean; it was to kill off the ticks and chiggers that might have gotten through your clothes and started looking for some nice warm spot to burrow in. If you didn't get them in time, next day you'd be nothing but a giant welt.

To see the actual places where I grew up, a car won't do. You need to go by pickup truck. Both the houses of my childhood are gone now, the Ollie Reed place and the Old Wes Jones place. All that's left of them are little flattened rises in the middle of overgrown meadows that used to be full of cotton and corn. But the landmarks are still there, like the big sweet gum tree. We used to take lunch in its shade, Mama and Daddy coming up from the fields they were working, me and the other children coming in from ours. The tree gave off a sap you could chew like gum.

Go down beyond the gum tree toward the bottom, and you're walking through what used to be our big stand of sugarcane. You can't see any traces of that anymore. But the pear tree is still heavy with fruit, even though it's hedged in by other trees that sprouted up after we left. Not far from there our old overflowing well is bubbling out a steady stream of water, the same as always. That was our main source at the Ollie Reed place. It was wonderful, clear water, which we appreciated a lot more after we moved to Wes Jones. But it was a good quarter mile from the house, which made hauling the buckets a hard task.

Off behind the well in a thicket is the old family cemetery where many of Mama's people are buried. It's uncared for now and overgrown. It's in the process of returning to nature. Right next to it is the remains of an even older cemetery, long abandoned even when I was a child. We think it was a burial ground of the Joneses. They were one of the early white families in Schaal and still big landowners by local standards when we farmed the land. We knew them all well, especially Miss May Dorsey, a Jones daughter who lived up the lane from us. Her boy Glenn Dean played with my brothers, and she and Mama helped each other out when babies were sick or other emergencies came up, which they did regularly.

By contrast with the overflowing well, our dug well near the house was shallow and brackish. At times the surface got a kind of green scum on it, and it wasn't all that unusual for the whole family to come down with stomach distress and diarrhea. The same was true for the Old Wes Jones place, where we moved when I was twelve. Wes Jones didn't even have a privy, though I suppressed that memory for years. But I do have a sharp recollection of the privy behind the Ollie Reed house. That place frightened me every time I had to use it. Especially the screw-worms that crawled around in there, big and fat as a small snake.

Whenever my mother's reading lessons got too confusing for me, I used to run and hide behind that privy. "Now you tell me," Mama would say, "what happens when you put that *e* after the word? What's that make it?" This is one of my first clear memories. I could read the word fine. I just had. It was "c-a-p, cap." But my four-year-old brain was having a hard time getting itself around the final *e* idea. Out of the corner of my eye I could see the switch in Mama's hand beginning to bounce a little. She'd tan the back of my legs with that if my progress slacked off too much. Mama's switching wasn't meant to hurt, but it stung enough so I wanted to avoid it. "I got to go, Mama. I got to go bad. I'll be right back." And I'd race out to the privy and stand behind it, not wanting to duck inside, because of the worms, but not wanting to go back to the house either. I'd wait it out as long as I could, hoping that she'd start doing something else and forget about the lesson. But she never would. "You got to learn your letters, honey, and your numbers. You've got to get a good start."

"You've got to get a good start!" I think she said that as often as she said prayers. Mama was a small, wiry woman, always smiling, always with a good word for everyone and a heartful of love. A wonderful, giving-of-herself kind of person. She never looked at the negative side of things, either then or until she passed last year at age eighty-three. She was always a sunny optimist, even when there was precious little to be optimistic about. Even when things were horrible, she always thought that she was just the luckiest woman in the world. "I'm so grateful all my children are healthy and nothing's wrong with them," she'd say. "I just feel rich."

Mama's name was Haller. She was born Reed, which became Jones when she and Daddy, Curtis Jones, got married secretly. She was eighteen, and he was nineteen, so they weren't children. But the families hadn't been told, much less asked. So it wasn't smooth. Mama was on the girls' basketball team at school, and the story goes that she came home on the bus in her basketball uniform. But instead of going inside to do her after-school chores she ran off in her shorts to meet Daddy and get to the preacher. Those who remember say that Haller's daddy, my grandpa Charlie Reed, was so mad he went looking for his new son-in-law with a shotgun. He calmed down later, though I always had a sense that Daddy's family might have been happier with the match than Mama's was.

In those days school went only part-time since all the students worked regularly on the farm. As a result, extremely few of them graduated, and all of them were older for their grade level than is common nowadays. Mama finished the eighth grade herself, which was pretty good for a black woman growing up in the southwestern corner of Arkansas in the first part of the century. And she had a tremendous determination that all her children were going to be educated. She didn't ease off any on the seven that came after me. But as her first I experienced that determination at its fiercest.

It wasn't that Mama had any particular aspirations for us, like becoming a doctor or lawyer or professor. Professions like that were outside our world. Going to college wasn't something that ever occurred to any of us. The only thing we ever saw people doing was work; I'm talking hard physical labor. The only time we ever saw anybody in a suit was in church. Everybody we knew was in overalls driving mules. But somehow Mama held tight to the conviction that if we ever wanted to "be something," we had better get educated.

"Being something" might have been on Mama's tongue a lot, but it wasn't something I ever particularly thought about. I did sometimes fantasize about becoming a store clerk. To be a clerk in a ten-cent store or a grocery store would have been a real improvement, particularly when the temperature in the fields got up around a hundred and the mosquitoes were swarming and the humidity made the air so thick you could all but see it. Days like that, being a clerk in some kind of cool, dim store seemed like it might be a good way to spend your life. Clerks didn't plow fields or weed furrows. They didn't chop cotton or strip cane or bale hay from sunup to sundown. The only problem was that no store clerk I had ever seen was black. Around Schaal, indoor work was white. Except for maids. Maids worked inside, but maid work didn't exactly seem like "being something."

By the time I was five I was well prepared for school. By then I was already a good reader, which allowed Mama to go to work on my sister Katie, who was two years younger than I. I had long outgrown the primer Mama used for lessons and had taken to reading the Bible, which was the other book in the house. My brother Chester, who's a Methodist minister now, tells everyone that the reason he went into the church is that the Bible was the only book we had around for him to read. It was my only book too, and though I didn't become a minister, more than once I've had people accuse me of preaching. I also pored over the weekly *Grit,* a farmers' newspaper out of Kansas that Daddy subscribed to. When I finally started first grade at Bright Star school, I was astonished to find I could always get some kind of book there, like *Grimm's Fairy Tales.* Not only that, but I could take it home and read at night after everything that had to get done had gotten done. I'd prop a blanket on the floor like a tent, put a coal-oil lamp under it, and curl up with Hansel and Gretel.

Katie and I slept in one bed in the second of our three rooms, where we were soon joined by our brothers Charles and Bernard. After that my parents took a little rest before they started having Chester, Beryl, Pat, and Phillip. Being the oldest automatically made me the work leader and the baby nurse. But I don't really remember ever taking care of Katie. I always felt like she was helping me, whereas Charles and Bernard and the others I was constantly looking after. Mama would have the new baby, and I'd have the rest.

Katie was my friend and companion in helping keep the house and farm going. I did whatever I could for my age, and Katie followed right behind me, doing everything she could: drag a bucket, scrub clothes, haul a little water from the well. In the morning we got up as soon as we heard Mama and Daddy stirring. Then we started in on the chores that had to get done before school time, first of all building the fire, then slopping the hogs.

Because water had to be brought up from a distance, we used it sparsely. Even the used dishwater got saved in a big five-gallon can by the back door, which was also where we threw all the leftover kitchen scraps. Whatever was in that can went for the hogs. Daddy also bought something called shorts, a kind of coarse reddish gray meal that we kept out in the smokehouse. Every morning first thing Katie and I would bring in a bagful of shorts and mix it up with the slops. Then she'd get on one side of the can and I'd get on the other. We'd both grab the handle, trying to get a little of the wooden middle of it so we wouldn't hurt our hands as much, and we'd carry and drag it out to the pen and pour it in the trough.

We might have had six or seven hogs in the pen, and while we were pouring, they would crowd in and start eating. They would be all around us, snuffling and grunting. Some of them must have weighed four hundred pounds, but big as they were, we didn't have any fear of them. You could push on them and they'd move. Hit them on the head and they'd back up.

The slop would never be enough, so we'd have to get a batch of dried corn from the barn and throw some of that to them too. I don't remember ever having too much of a personal relationship with pigs. We had some cows we had more of a friendship with, but not pigs.

Once the hogs were done, the cows had to be milked. Oftentimes we'd have to go get them from the pasture and bring them down into the barn. Though I don't remember exactly, I think my aunts and uncles on my mother's side must have taught me how to milk. Grandpa Charlie Reed owned lots of cows, and he and his children milked them. They sold milk and cream. My uncles Slim and Bone and Dr. Tom and Aunt Suzy and Uncle Buh—Buddy—would milk twenty or thirty cows twice a day.

At our house we had only four or five cows. Katie and I would go get them with a little stick and herd them in. Small as we were, there was no problem. Cows herd pretty easily. We'd get them into the barn, then let their calves in to them so they could suck a little. The calves' sucking made the milk let down into the teats. When the calves had sucked some, we'd put a rope around them and pull them over to the fence, where we tied them up so they couldn't get back at the cows. Then we could start milking. Without the calves stimulating the let-down, milking would have been too hard for us. But once the milk came down, it was easy as pie. All it needed was gentle pulling. Besides, if you did it too hard, the cow would kick you. We were always careful not to take all the milk, though. You had to leave some for the calves after.

We milked those cows every day, but I never did become a champion milker. I always held my bucket with one hand while I milked with the other. I was afraid to put the bucket on the ground because I thought the cow might kick it over. So I was never brave enough to use both hands and go full speed, the way Aunt Suzy and Uncle Buh taught me to do.

When we were finished milking, we hauled the big milk canister back in the house and strained it. We used a clean sheet for that, to make sure that any extraneous material wasn't in there. After we strained it, we covered it up in what we called the milk bucket and set it out on the back porch to clabber— that is, to ferment. We'd let it clabber; then we'd churn butter and buttermilk later on. Regular milk would go bad in a day, but buttermilk kept.

By the time we were finished chores the sky would be lightening and Mama would have breakfast ready. Usually she'd make rice and biscuits, ham or salt meat, and always something sweet, like molasses bread and jam. She'd cook enough for breakfast and lunch both. Then we'd all sit down at the big table and say grace. "Good Lord, we thank Thee for the blessings we are about to receive for the nourishment and strength of our bodies, for Christ's sake. Amen."

Just in front of our house was a little creek branch. When I started school at Bright Star, I'd wait for the kids from the four or five houses below us to come by, maybe six of us all together.

The branch crossed the road, and Daddy used to lay down planks over it. But every time it rained the branch would pool and the planks would wash away. So we'd wade it or jump. Either way everybody's shoes would get sopped, and we'd walk to school with wet feet.

I always walked with Clara Dean Davis, who was my best friend and in the same grade as I was. We'd take the muddy trail a couple of miles through the woods until we reached the main road, talking all the way. Usually it was about dolls or what we were doing in school or the houses we'd have when we grew up. Nice, big houses. By that we meant bigger than the unpainted three-room shacks we both lived in. By nice we thought about windows that weren't broken and covered with cardboard or a roof that didn't leak in a dozen places. We didn't dream of electricity. We didn't know about it, so we didn't miss it. Nobody had electricity, or indoor plumbing either. Neither of us had seen a real bathtub.

Bright Star was really just a wide place in the road. There was a store and a pasture across the road that the men kept cleared so they could play baseball on Saturday afternoons. Then there was Bright Star elementary, where we went. Bright Star elementary was painted white. It had two rooms and a kind of recessed alcove where the front door was that we could stand under if it rained during lunch or recess. In the middle of the room was a potbellied stove. All the kids sat on long wooden benches. There were no desks, just benches. I'm pretty certain the white schools had desks at that time, given the way things were. But we worked on our laps on big sheets of paper we'd tear off a tablet.

Our teacher, Miss Ulistine Brown, taught a roomful of kids who might have ranged in age from five to thirteen. Since we didn't have workbooks, she'd write out our lessons on the board and we'd copy them on to our paper. She would have one group doing numbers, another writing, and a third doing something else—all at the same time. Thinking back on it, I know that classroom must have been a noisy place, but I don't remember any of us noticing. When you lived in a house where there might be four or eight or ten children, there wasn't all that much difference.

Shortly after I got home from school each day, we'd eat supper. Daddy would come in from working, and we'd all sit down around the long kitchen table. Everybody always ate together, no matter what. Later on, when I had my own family, that was still important to me. But back then it was survival. If you had eight kids and you were fixing three meals a day, no one had any choice. If you fixed it and someone wasn't there to eat, that person didn't get any. So you never had a problem getting people to the table. It was all served family style in big bowls: the peas and butter beans and fried corn and squash and ham and whatever else was ready in the garden or Daddy had hunted, all depending on the season.

I'd talk while we ate, about what had happened in school, what I had learned, or who might have done what to whom. Katie and Charles and the others would be babbling too. But it was mainly Mama who carried the conversation with us. Daddy mostly talked when someone got out of hand. Even then he'd limit himself to something like "Didn't y'all hear your mother?" I never had the feeling that he wasn't interested in us; he just wasn't given to words. The only real talking he was going to do was when you came in from working a section of field. Then he'd ask how it went, or how much you had got chopped, or if you had any trouble with the mule. It was not what you would call an actual conversation per se.

The fact was that Daddy was consumed by work. Mama labored side by side with him in the fields, but she also took care of the garden and the cooking and the house and of course the baby. The eight of us were spread out over eighteen years, which meant she was either pregnant or nursing for most of that time. But Daddy's life was on the land. From spring through fall he was always plowing, planting, chopping, picking, cutting, or baling. In the winter he hunted and trapped, raccoon mainly, but also possum and squirrel and wild mink.

Sometimes he and a few of his friends would get their dogs together and go after a fox. But his serious hunting he did by himself, and that was most of the time. Hunting for Daddy was work. Selling hides to Sears and Montgomery Ward was one of the few cash-money sources he had. He'd hunt coons with the dogs he bought from a breeder in Paducah, Kentucky, all of them with papers. He prided himself on those dogs. Most people we knew had dogs that were maybe half hunting dog, half stray mongrel. But for Daddy a good coon dog was an investment. His sweat was going mainly into sharecropping other people's land, which was what we were doing on the Old Wes Jones place. But he used the raccoon money to start buying up land for himself, a little section at a time. It took years, but eventually he had eighty acres of his own, most all of it bought with coonskins.

With that driving him, Daddy was out in the woods the whole winter, mainly at night, which is when you hunt raccoons. The dogs would pick up a scent, chase the coon down, and tree him, Daddy following close behind. Then he'd shine his flashlight up in the tree, catch the gleam in the coon's eyes, and shoot him.

When he got home, he skinned the coons and stretched the hides. I helped with the stretching and sometimes with the skinning, which had to be done carefully so the hide wouldn't be marked. You didn't want to touch the back part, so you cut them across the forepaws, straight down the underside, then up across the back paws. You skin out from the head and around the paws. Then you stretch it out. We'd sit in front of the fireplace and nail the hides up on boards using these tiny nails. We'd stretch and pull. I handed him the tacks, and he knocked them in.

Once he had gotten the skin off, Daddy would give the raccoon to Mama to cook, and I helped with that too. First we removed the musk glands; then we put the coon whole into salted water and parboiled it, just let him bleach out until he got tender. Then we took him out, arranged sweet potatoes all around, and baked him in the oven. Mama made the best raccoon in the world. It had a distinctive taste, like a cross between deer and turkey. It's all red meat, like beef, and coarse like beef, but laid out like rabbit. You could sell the raccoon meat in addition to the hide. But mainly we ate it ourselves. In the winter it was probably our primary source of meat, along with possum. We baked possum too, more or less the same way.

Daddy also hunted hogs. Like almost everyone else, he let some of his hogs run loose. He put his mark on them, an underbit in both ears and the right ear cropped. Then he set them free in the bottom, where we didn't have to feed them. They foraged for themselves down there, living mainly off the acorns.

Some of them just didn't survive, and some of them would get into people's crops in the summer. When that happened, he'd have to hunt them down then, and often they'd get too hot and just die. But usually he hunted hogs in the fall, when it was cool. His dogs would track them and chase them down until they could bay them somewhere. They'd be snapping and yapping, keeping the hogs' attention while Daddy found a spot where he could rope them with his lariat. Ordinarily he went after the two-year-olds, but some of those hogs would stay uncaught year after year and truly turn wild. Once in a while he lost a dog to them. Their tusks were sharp as razors, and they could just lay a dog open so his intestines would fall out.

Aside from the occasional fox hunts with his cronies, Daddy's one real pleasure was baseball. Saturdays most folks would try to quit work around noon. That was the day the men played baseball on the field they kept cleared across from the Bright Star store. As many people as could make it would go up to watch, especially teenagers, who were glad for a chance to flirt and hang out with their friends. Daddy played catcher and some first base. His arm was so strong he could rifle a man out at second without budging off his squat. Even today Uncle Reva and Uncle Gus will swear he was good enough to have played in the professional Negro Leagues. That isn't just their opinion. Lots of folks used to say that. Daddy was powerfully built, six feet, 190 pounds, and muscular. He had big-league speed and could hit a mile.

All the towns around had teams: Mineral Springs, Tollette, Brownstown, Okay. They played each other, and they played the different sawmill teams, which always had ringers. The mills used to vie with one another to hire the best ballplayers. The Schaal team traveled too, in a rickety caravan of maybe a couple of Model As and somebody's makeshift truck. They went to places as far as Hope and Broken Bow, Oklahoma, and Springhill, Louisiana. Once they played a white team from Texarkana and whipped them. Daddy was known as a first-class farmer, hunter, hog raiser, and cattleman. But baseball was where he really shone.

Playing baseball was a relief from the never-ending work and considerable anxiety Daddy had to live with. He and Mama didn't show their worries much. But I think there was a kind of background of fear in their lives, like there is for farmers generally, except worse because we lived so near the brink. Things happened that you couldn't control, that could turn all your work to nothing. Things like cotton worm and drought and floods, when Mine Creek or the Saline River overflowed and covered the corn up to the top tassles. Things that overwhelmed you, like the tornadoes that would rip down swaths of trees like a bulldozer.

Often we had some warning of tornadoes. There was a white lady, Miss Hosey, who lived across from where Mama and Daddy lived till recently, which is maybe a mile from where the Ollie Reed place used to be. Miss Hosey had a kind of sixth sense for tornadoes. When she felt one coming, she got her big dinner bell and clanged it hard as she could. You'd hear her bell a mile away; then after a bit you'd hear other bells joining in. Every family had a bell, and since no one owned a watch, the bells rang out every day to call people in for lunch and dinner. Nobody paid any attention to anyone else's lunch or dinner bells. But if a bell rang any other time, it meant emergency. Then your heart would start racing, and you ran to get your own bell and ring it, to warn others. You couldn't hear a bell without feeling you had to drop everything and start ringing. The whole countryside would be echoing with bells.

They rang for fires, and they rang whenever someone died. But when a bell sounded down from Miss Hosey's direction, you could be pretty certain it was a tornado coming. Most often in tornado weather we were already inside the house, though that was no protection. Houses tended to be so poorly built that they'd get blown down or just splintered, with their pieces scattered across the countryside. A lot of people had tornado cellars they'd get down into. We didn't. Instead we'd all get into the hall and lie down on the floor with a quilt over us, our hands over our eyes to protect them from things that might come flying.

Even more fearful than tornadoes, though in a different way, were the locusts that showed up every couple of years. We knew by word of mouth when the locusts were coming. Somebody would report that they had been spotted down in Tollette, which immediately got everybody in Schaal nervous. After that people watched and waited. Then neighbors started saying that they had been seen in Mr. Dillard's cornfields yesterday or that they were swarming in the bottoms. By that time we were praying hard that they would bypass us. Not necessarily that they would land on somebody else's field, but at least that they wouldn't land on ours.

Sometimes we would see only a sprinkling of them on the edges of the pasture. But other times it was like something out of the Bible. They'd look like a black horror coming through the sky, making a kind of ungodly zinging noise. Once you heard that noise, you never forgot it. Then they'd settle and start eating, swarms of them just everywhere, and you'd hear this horrible chopping sound, rustling and chopping. When I was visiting my folks down there a couple of years ago, I heard it again; it set my teeth right on edge. Two or three days and they could devour the entire cotton crop we had chopped and fertilized and worked so hard on. We didn't know anything to do about it, no more than anyone else. All you could do was watch.

I felt deeply afraid at times like that, overwhelmed by what was happening. So did my sisters and brothers. But I'm sure Mama and Daddy were more in despair than we we were. Cotton was our cash crop. That's what gave us most of whatever money we were able to get in a year. Of course I didn't appreciate the significance of that quite as much as I do now, and somehow children feel their parents will always find a way. Somehow things will be all right. But scenes like that must have just knotted their insides with fear.

As I got older, I understood it better. I came to recognize the hurt in Mama's eyes when we were riding headlong into some calamity. But she was always the one comforting everybody else, giving strength to us at those critical junctures when the cows got something and died or the hogs died or drowned in the floods and we lost the crops. These didn't happen all the time. But every once in a while they hit. "It's going to be all right," she'd say, almost like a refrain. So many times I heard, "Curtis, it's going to be all right. We'll make it. We'll make it." The house might be burning down around our ears, but she'd be sure that we were "going to be all right." And bad as the situation might seem, there was nothing hollow in her words. She was absolutely convinced that in the end the good Lord would take care of her. She believed it. And because she did, we did.

———

One winter Bernard got sick. First he started complaining that his stomach hurt him, which nobody paid that much attention to. Stomach ailments weren't exactly uncommon in our house. It could have been something in the water, or maybe he had eaten some green apples, which was a favorite explanation for stomachaches. I didn't doubt that he really might have eaten some green apples. Bern was about the most rambunctious four-year-old you could ever imagine, always getting into a mess or fighting with Charles or climbing on things. You could tell him not to eat green apples a hundred times and he'd go and eat the first one he could locate. But then he started running a fever, and nothing Mama gave him would stay down. After he started throwing up, he wouldn't take anything at all. He just lay there with his eyes wide open, saying, "My stomach hurts."

That night I listened to Bernard whining softly and grunting like a little pig in the bed he shared with Charles across the room from Katie and me. "Unh, unh, unh," all night long. Next day his stomach started to swell up. Mama had put a kind of loose gown on him, probably somebody's shirt, and I sat next to him on the bed, sponging him off, trying to get the fever to go down. I mopped his forehead and his chest and his skinny little legs. But it wasn't helping. It looked to me like his stomach was bulging out. When I touched it, it was hard as a rock. Mama kept coming in from the kitchen to look. "Oh, my," she said. "We can't just let him lay there like this. Oh, my, we just got to get my baby to the doctor."

I was nine then, and that was the first I had ever heard Mama say anything about going to a doctor. In Schaal, if somebody got sick or hurt, people didn't necessarily associate that with going to doctors. Doctors cost money, and for the most part Schaal didn't run on a money economy. Besides, the nearest one was a white doctor twelve miles away. That meant a day there and back if you didn't have a car, which almost no one did. So that twelve miles might as well have been a thousand.

I had watched my aunt Mary die of meningitis, her neck stretched out and her back arched up. Later, my grandpa Charlie Reed died of appendicitis. Neither of them saw a doctor. No more than Mama had when she had her babies or my schoolmate little Val Belcher had when he was kicked in the head by a mule at the age of four and left palsied and crippled. The beginning and end of my understanding on the subject were that if you got sick or something happened to you, either you pulled through or you died. There wasn't much else.

So when Daddy came in from hunting that night, I was surprised to hear Mama tell him he had to take Bernard to the doctor. "Well," said Daddy. I could tell he wasn't prepared for what Mama had said and he needed to think about it. Daddy might have respected Mama most often, but he didn't always worry too much about doing what she said to do. But Mama was determined to save Bernard if she could. "Curtis," she said, "if this child makes it through till morning, you have got to take him."

I don't know what Mama and Daddy thought, but I guessed

that Bernard was probably going to die that night. He was usually such a chatterbox, but now he wasn't saying a word. All night long I listened in the dark. I could make out Charles's regular breathing, but there was no sound from Bernard, except for a little grunt every now and then.

The next morning when I woke up and went over to look, Bernard wasn't moving. But I could feel his chest rising and falling, and he grunted a couple of times, though much softer now than last night. Daddy was already out in the lot getting the mule ready, and Mama was at the stove cooking something up for him. It was obvious she wasn't thinking about a thing except getting him and Bernard off. After Daddy ate, he put on his hunting coat, the heavy brown one with the corduroy collar and all the little pockets for his shotgun shells. Then he held a blanket while Mama picked Bernard up and wrapped him into it. When Daddy took him, Bernard's head fell back, and he winced from the pull on his swollen stomach. "You got to hold his head up, Curtis," said Mama. "Hold his head up so he don't hurt so bad."

I watched Daddy go out and get on the mule. It looked like he had rigged up something in front of the saddle to rest Bernard on while they were riding. Then Mama and I stood and watched as he turned the mule around and went across the branch. We watched them pass the house up the road where Miss Grace and Mr. Sleety lived and go on around the bend. Then they disappeared behind the cottonwoods.

———

It wasn't till late at night that we heard the mule come back. When we went out to see, there was Daddy sitting on Old Jim holding Bernard in his arms, still bundled up in the blanket. Bernard looked the same as when he had left, huge-eyed and silent as death. But when we took the blanket off, I saw a big red tube sticking out of his stomach. The doctor had told Daddy Bernard's appendix had burst. He put the big red tube in there to drain the poison out of him. Then he sent them home. There were no hospitals around there for any black children.

Chapter 2

What I Saw

❧❧❧

Here's a conversation I had with a friend of mine who was asking about how I grew up. I was describing how one time I slipped in the yard and cut my foot on a broken jar. It was a bad gash, from my big toe along the sole of my foot almost to the heel. I still have the scar from it. I was telling him about how my mother treated it with coal oil. My friend said, "I've never heard of coal oil. What's coal oil?"

I said, "Coal oil. Coal oil. It's oil that you burn, like kerosene."

MY FRIEND: You mean that you used in lamps? This was the closest you had to an antiseptic?
ME: Oh, we used it all the time.
MY FRIEND: This was your home remedy? Coal oil?
ME: Yeah. Coal oil. It's c-o-a-l o-i-l. Coal oil.
MY FRIEND: What if somebody had a headache? Did you have any aspirin around the house?
ME: No, we never heard of aspirin.

Ask my mother how she treated a fever and she'd have to think a minute. Then she'd remember that she used to boil jimsonweed tea, which you had to let steep awhile. Or you could make up a poultice of jimsonweed and vinegar, put it on the patient's forehead, and let him sweat the fever out. She'd tell you she used mullen leaf tea for colds, though you could also try horehound. For hives you steamed red onion and catnip; for worms you gave a mixture of sugar and turpentine. Calamus root was good for stomach problems; just scrape the root and chew.

She'd be smiling while she told you this. It's not just that she knew you'd think these were quaint home remedies that might not be all that helpful. It's that she knew it too. She knew it back when she was using them on us. Jimsonweed and horehound were the equivalent of saying, "Oh, Lord, there's nothing I can do about this, but I've at least got to try something rather than just sit here." In reality, we were in God's hands, and she knew it.

Her psychology, which was also Daddy's, grew out of her knowing that every day could and very likely would bring some kind of crisis. Katie would get hit in the head with a grubbing hoe. I would lay my foot open. Daddy would get slashed by some boar he was after. Somebody would step on a rusty nail or get bitten by a water moccasin. Something was going to happen for sure.

When it did, you were on your own. You weren't going to go up to the hospital emergency room and get it fixed. There wasn't any hospital. You weren't going to make an appointment to go see your family doctor. You didn't have a doctor. If Chester stepped on a nail, you put coal oil on it and prayed that this wasn't the nail that was going to give him lockjaw. If Pat was attacked by a strange dog, you waited to see if that dog had had rabies in its bite. And your anxiety level shot right up. You weren't calm. Because you knew people who had died grinning with tetanus or deranged with hydrophobia.

The way you survived in those circumstances was by living each day by faith in God. That was your shield against the idea that life is mostly just disasters and tragedies. When you have faith, you see it differently. You understand that even apparent tragedies can be for the better one way or another. Faith gives you a way to search for the positive in what might otherwise overwhelm you with negatives. All of us picked up our faith from Mama. We got it by growing up the way we did and, more important, by being around her, seeing her on her knees. "Just pray," she said. "Ask God and pray."

My brother Chester, the minister, says he used to think Mama's praying was just a kind of passive acceptance, something you might do to pacify yourself. But eventually he understood it wasn't that. When Mama talked to God, it was active. She would get down on her knees and pray about whatever was troubling her until some kind of solution or answer began to come out of it. She knew it was painful. She knew that it was hard and that she didn't understand it. But she also knew that her good Lord would take care of her. In many ways I'm different from my mother. I've been to college and medical school and postgraduate school. But we share a lot too. She gave me and all the rest of us faith.

Mama didn't talk much about religion; she just lived it. Her piety wasn't for show. Nor did she talk about other people's faith or whether they had it or not. She didn't even necessarily make it to church each and every Sunday, even though she made sure all the children did.

Our church, Tabernacle Methodist, was a mile and a half down the road. It was a little white one-room church, built on high brick blocks with concrete steps going up to double doors. It used to be up on a lovely hill, though they've moved it now. The children would go to Sunday school first for Bible lessons, and after that would be services. Daddy would come in and take a seat with the deacons, and Mama would sit near the back. Tabernacle Methodist was too small to have its own pastor, but a preacher would come twice a month. The other two Sundays everyone would go over to Bright Star Baptist. The Baptists didn't have their own minister either, so their part-time preacher arranged with our part-time preacher to share the load. There might have been some doctrinal differences between the two, but if there were, neither of them ever mentioned it.

Most often people would bring baskets of food to church, and after service everyone would set the food outside on a table under the oak tree and there'd be a potluck picnic. That was dinner on the ground, getting together and sharing. That was pretty much the way people acted outside church too. Nobody thought twice about these things. You'd plant a big garden and somebody would come by and want something. They never asked. You'd just hear, "Oh, Haller, your greens are ready."

"Oh, yeah?" Mama would shout back. "Here, get your sack. Go out and get you some."

Everybody did that. In recent years my mother's biggest concern was that she didn't have anything to give to anybody because she couldn't raise her garden anymore. I'd say, "Mama, for sixty, seventy years you had a garden, and you gave corn and peas and beans and potatoes. And everybody came by, and you gave them a jar of this and a jar of that."

And she'd say, "Oh, everybody's so good to Mama. They just bring me all kinds of stuff."

She'd want to can peaches. "I need to can me some peaches," she'd say.

We'd tell her, "Mama, we'll buy you some peaches. It's cheaper to buy them."

She'd say, "Well, I just need some canned peaches because my children might come by, and I can't give them any home-canned peaches."

So we'd go get her some peaches and help get them ready so she could can some peaches. The last time she did that Chester said she was so tired she couldn't get up. But she canned them. You could never tell when somebody might stop by and need something.

It often surprises people when I tell them that this feeling of neighborliness and sharing wasn't limited to the black families in Schaal. I don't mean to say that the idea of equality was in the air while I was growing up. It wasn't. But neither were the anger and resentment between the races that existed in some other parts of Arkansas and the South. One reason may have been that Schaal was west of the Mississippi Delta, outside the historical culture of plantations and large-scale slavery. In our corner of the state relations had probably always been more personal. We didn't go to school and church with the white kids, which were big things, of course. But we played together, and many of our parents were in the habit of helping each other out. In those parts you weren't likely to scorn neighbors, whatever their color.

The white lady who lived across the road from us was Miss Young. She was always helping Mama, bringing her things and lending a hand when it was needed. If she was sick, you could find Mama over there washing her clothes and cleaning her house. Neighbors just felt they had a responsibility to take care of the neighbors.

That was also true of Miss May Dorsey, the Jones daughter who lived at the end of the lane who used to come wash clothes and cook when Mama had one of her difficult childbirths. May Dorsey has known me my entire life. When I started doing well in school and showing some ability, she was as proud of me as could be. The vocabulary she used back then would not pass muster now. "Yeah," she'd say, bragging about some school prize I might have won, "that's my little nigger girl." But there wasn't a drop of meanness or disrespect involved; she was just speaking the language of the times. She made it clear back then that she was proud to know me, and she has never lost her affection. Even now she and her son and two daughters will come up to Little Rock to visit. They think they need to. It's important to them, and it means a lot to me.

It wasn't any different with the men than with the women. My father was very involved with the local white farmers. They would exchange equipment and help each other out. If someone was in trouble and had a big hayfield that needed cutting, my dad and the others would all go and take their machines and do that farmer's haying for him.

Of course around Schaal the ties that bound people went beyond just neighborliness. Mama was the first of thirteen children; Daddy was the first of seventeen. Grandpa Charlie Reed had been one of twenty-six. In those days before easy mobility people tended to stay where they were. As a result, the Schaal area was jumping with Turners and Adamses and Reeds and Joneses, all of them our relations.

My mother's people, the Reeds, had been there a long time, from slave days as far as anyone can remember. Daddy's were later arrivals. I knew his grandmother well, my great-grandmother Minerva. She had long, straight silver hair, high cheekbones, and light, almost white skin. There was no question about her Indian ancestry, though her exact origins weren't completely clear. One story I've heard is that she came to Arkansas by wagon train from South Carolina. The more common account in the family is that she was a Choctaw from the Indian Territory in Oklahoma who married a former slave there and drifted east across the Arkansas border.

When I knew Minerva, she was quite old. She lived by herself in Hickory Grove, about twenty miles from Schaal, but she used to visit us every once in a while. She'd arrive in a wagon pulled by two horses, always with a great clatter. As soon as she got down, she'd start in hugging and kissing everyone in sight, me especially. Since I was her first great-grandchild, I got special attention. "Oh"—she'd laugh—"don't mind me. Your old granny's just crazy."

Her daughter was Daddy's mother, Minnie Jones, for whom I was named. It wasn't until college that I changed my name from Minnie Lee to Minnie Joycelyn, then just Joycelyn, which I took from a peppermint candy I was fond of. Mainly I wanted to be my own person. Before that I was Minnie, or Little Min (my grandmother being Big Min), or Mint, which is what my father called me. To most people in Schaal I'm still Minnie. As Grandma Minnie got older, she looked more and more like Minerva. Her straight black hair grew silver, and her cheekbones became more and more prominent. My dad too has an Indian cast of features and hair that's more Indian than African.

Minnie Jones was a character, a slim, beautiful, feisty woman, always upbeat, always positive, which was probably one of the reasons she and Mama got on so well. They had a lot in common. Unlike Mama, though, Grandma Minnie never spent much time working the fields. She didn't like field work at all and went to lengths to avoid it. She always thought it was funny, the tricks she played on Grandpa. She'd tell him she didn't feel well and had to stay home. Then, as soon as he was out of the house, she'd hitch up the wagon and go fishing all day. More than once I was with her when we had to tear out of the fishing hole so she could get home and start cooking dinner before everybody got back from work.

Minnie's husband, my grandpa Charlie Jones, was a handsome man with a mysterious past. He was from Louisiana originally, a woodsman and logroller who had floated logs down the Mississippi. But Jones wasn't his name then. The story whispered around the family was that he had gotten into some kind of trouble while logging on the Ouachita River. No one ever speculated out loud on what the trouble might have been. But it was bad enough so that he had himself snuck out of there, traveling in a pine coffin like a corpse in a wagon driven by a friend. Schaal was where he ended up, under the name of Charlie Jones. The place must have suited him. It was a backwater where people didn't get too inquisitive about someone else's history. And there was plenty of work. At the turn of the century the GN&A Railroad was laying track from Nashville to Ashdown, and lumberjacks and woodworkers were in heavy demand.

I saw both sets of grandparents often—Elnora and Charlie Reed as well as Minnie and Charlie Jones. Many weekends there'd be a major gathering of the family at one place or another, with what might be dozens of aunts and uncles and cousins. Grandma Minnie or Elnora would put on a great big meal, and everyone would bring children and dogs. Even after the children were married and gone, they still came back for those get-togethers.

While the adults gabbed and laughed and prepared food, the kids played ball or jacks or marbles. Somebody would always put together a seesaw, setting a long plank over whatever was around that could be used for the center. I played, but more often I tended to go off somewhere and read. Either that or go talk to my aunt **Annie**, who was five or six years older than I was. There were few enough moments in my life when there wasn't any work to do or children to tend, so when one came along, I grabbed it.

They had a lot of folks to feed at these things, and the food was plentiful, three or four different kinds of smoked meats, corn bread, sourdough biscuits, beans cooked with ham bones, corn on the cob, lots of sweet potatoes and squash, peas of different kinds—whippoorwill, black-eyed peas, purple hulled peas, crowder peas, and plenty of hot sweet chow-chow to go alongside. I may not have always had exactly what I wanted to eat, but the one thing that I don't ever remember being is hungry.

The drinks were tea and lemonade mainly. I don't ever recall very much liquor being drunk in my family. It's funny, you read memoirs and biographies from the South, and it's not unusual to find drinking and family violence. But I don't remember anybody that drank very much at all. I do remember that Uncle Slim made and sold bootleg, but even he didn't drink it. At our get-togethers the men weren't sucking down beers or nipping at bottles. They may have had a little bit to drink, but I don't recall anybody ever getting drunk.

There wasn't any alcoholism. Nor was there ever any talk of men beating their wives, or of separations or divorce either. If I look at my aunts and uncles, I don't remember ever having one that didn't continue to be an aunt or an uncle. That's true of both sides, among the whole considerable number of them. The one divorce I can think of is my sister Beryl, who's sixth in line. She and her husband, Elijah, divorced after their four children were fairly grown up. Elijah had a stroke recently, and right now Beryl's deciding if she is going to take him back in and take care of him. They stayed friends even after they separated.

These husbands and wives weren't given to demonstrating their affection in public, but you had the definite feeling that they cared. There was warmth there. They felt responsible for each other, which was a good thing, because they had a lot of work to do together.

One of my first clear memories is of Mama teaching me to read with her switch. This is another, from about the same time frame. I'm in the back of the wagon with Katie, sitting on a quilt. There are some other things in the wagon bed with us, a plow and a crosstie. Daddy's up front driving the mule, and the three of us are on our way out to the fields to work together. I don't remember having gone out to work with him before, so this is probably my first time. I'm excited.

Mama isn't along, which must mean that she's either having a baby or she just had one. Katie is about two and a half, so the baby must be our new brother Charles. That puts us in April 1938, which makes me four and a half. Today Katie and I are going to help Daddy plant corn.

Next thing I know we're standing out in the field and Daddy's showing me the furrows he's started making with the plow. He's bending down, pointing out what's open furrow and what isn't. He does this very gently and precisely, as if he's talking to a little child, which of course he is. I've got the corn seeds in a square pouch that's hanging over my shoulder. The idea is that I'm supposed to drop the seeds straight along the furrows while Daddy finishes plowing. Then he's going to harness the crosstie to the mule and drag it over the rows I've planted to cover the seeds up. The pouch is making me feel very grown up. I've seen Mama wearing it many times. It feels coarse to the touch, though not as coarse as a croaker sack does.

After that things turn anxious. Daddy's off with the mule somewhere, and I'm staring at the ground, trying to figure out where the furrow is. In my memory I can see that field as clearly as if I were standing in it right now. And I still can't tell what is furrow from what isn't. I'm sure they're there, as straight as an arrow. But you don't plow deep for corn, and to my four-and-a-half-year-old eyes it all just looks like a big field of plowed dirt.

I'm really upset. I want to help Daddy so badly, but I just can't make out where to drop the seed corn. Instead I'm kind of scattering it around aimlessly, which I know can't be right. I'm so frustrated I could stamp. Daddy brought me out here to make the work go faster, which I know is important to him even if I couldn't tell you why. And now I'm messing up.

The last bit of this memory is that Daddy came over again. He must have seen what was happening. He may have tried to explain it again, but if he did, it didn't do any good. I still couldn't make out those rows. Finally he took the seed bag off my shoulder and said, "Mint, why don't y'all go back up there and sit in the wagon." I was hurt and bothered. I understood that what I had done had made him go slower instead of faster. And I just needed so much to help him with that field.

Later on I got better at it. Then before long Katie started working with me, doing whatever I was doing. We'd be working in one place while Mama and Daddy were off working someplace else. When Charles came along, we took care of him and worked at the same time, until he got old enough to toddle along behind us. Then it was Bernard and after a while Chester, Beryl, Pat, and Phillip.

From the time I was about five until I left home I was head of that work crew. It was a strange thing, I always felt I had to make sure that we had done enough work so that Daddy wouldn't be upset. Not that he did get upset much. He didn't have to. With him you understood what his expectations were, and you wanted to get them done. You just did. Daddy was one of those people with natural authority. He didn't use threats or force; he just imposed himself on the work and on everybody who was working around him.

I used to think that was just my impression, a daughter reacting to her father. But adults who knew him responded the same way. "He could put all of the accent where it needed to be when it needed to be there," is the way my husband, Oliver, describes it. "He told you where it was and how it was. You just didn't want to get on the wrong side of Mr. Curtis."

I say it was strange, because my dad wasn't a traditional disciplinarian. He told me once that his father used to hit them and that he had promised himself he was never going to do that to his children. Mama would take a switch to you at times, but he never did. The one time he came close sticks in my mind as vividly as I'm sure it does with my sisters and brothers.

I don't even remember what it was about, but we must have done something awful. He told us to cut switches and wait for him at the lot gate while he got done whatever he was getting done. "Go get 'em," he said. We cut our switches from what we called the toothbrush tree, a kind of ash tree with supple branches. Then we stood there in a line holding them, if you can picture that. We stood at that gate for what seemed like hours, though it probably wasn't more than ten or twenty minutes. When Daddy got through with what he was doing, he walked toward us, then walked right on by and went into the house. He didn't say a word. It was as if we weren't even there. After a while we came on in the house ourselves, very quietly. Then we sat around being nervous until Mama said it was time to go to bed.

I didn't have Daddy's temperament when it came to getting people to work. I didn't have Mama's either. She'd catch flies with sugar; I pushed. My mother says I had a temper, that I'd tell them a time or two, then I'd be all over them. Chester remembers it more or less the same way. We were talking about this once, and he brought up a time when I must have gotten to be too much for him. He yelled—this is his memory now— "You ain't my mama!"

And I said, "Well, I don't care. Just you do it."

"You'd whup us," he says. And once or twice I might have.

The four oldest of us worked together on our own for years, stripping cane, chopping sprouts, chopping cotton, picking cotton. We did everything there was to do. Growing cotton, you plant four or five times as many seeds as you need to make sure you have a good stand. Then what you have to do is to go through with a hoe and thin it out. Make the plants a hoe length apart, two and at the most three plants at each interval. That's chopping cotton. Sometimes you have to go back and chop it a second time.

Chopping cotton wasn't bad. Picking cotton was something

else. Picking cotton, you were stooped over all day long, dragging a heavy cotton sack behind you. From the time I was twelve my back always hurt. Later on we found out I had disk problems. I wasn't the only one. Five of my brothers and sisters had disk surgery when they were adults. I hurt so much I would get down and crawl on my knees. A lot of people did that. There were even knee pads made of leather with cushioning inside, though unfortunately we didn't have them.

Whoever Mama's newest baby was at any particular time, that was my responsibility too. So whatever field we happened to be working, I'd take the baby along and spread out a pallet under the nearest shade tree. That way I could always see him (or her) or at least hear if he started to cry.

The problem was snakes. Where we lived there were a lot of snakes, some of them really nasty—water moccasins, copperheads, and rattlesnakes. But fortunately we had Old Don, our big bulldog. Old Don was dark brown with white blotches and a bobbed tail. Like most bulldogs, he was just as mild as could be. But he was also a killer. Unlike Daddy's hunting dogs, he had a powerful protective instinct. Sometimes the hunting dogs would be out in the fields with us too. But if they felt like they wanted to go exploring off in the woods, they would just go. You had no sense that they would stay there, no matter what you might tell them. But you could tell Old Don to stay with the baby, and he knew it was his job to watch over whatever might be going on around that quilt. Don would kill any snake that came near, the same as he did in the yard around the house. He'd get it and break its neck. If the baby tried to crawl off the quilt, he'd pull him right back on by his diaper.

Don lived eighteen years, until he was finally killed in one of Daddy's hog hunts. That was the heart of the time when we were all growing up. He's there in my earliest memories, and he didn't die until after I left home. He let us ride on his back, and he kept us safe. All of us felt that somehow Old Don would take care of us, regardless. If a bear had suddenly appeared, we would have figured that Old Don could handle it. It was like having a personal guardian.

Snakes are one of my two phobias (the other is getting caught in an enclosed place). Even having Old Don around didn't alleviate my fear of snakes much. I was pretty sure snakes lived under our house, way under where Don couldn't get at them. Some of our floorboards had cracks in them almost wide enough to fall through. You could look down into the dark and think about some big snake slithering up into the house at night while you were sleeping. Snakes have a peculiar smell about them, a kind of rich, musty odor. I used to think I could smell them down there.

———

Way out in the bottom was a pond we called the Old Friday fishing hole, and just beyond that lay one of Daddy's big cotton patches. This place was about half a mile from the overflowing well, which meant that if you wanted a drink of water, you had to walk over a mile there and back. One day we were chopping cotton in that field, and for some reason I don't remember it was important to get the whole thing done right then. We worked all afternoon in one-hundred-plus-degree weather, and hot as it was, we didn't want to take the time to quit for a hike up to the well.

I was really chopping hard so we could get finished, and I was sweating profusely, losing lots of water and probably lots of salt too. When we finally did get through and made it up to the well, my mouth was parched so dry my tongue was cleaving to my palate. Looking back, I know I was severely dehydrated. Then all I knew was that I was thirstier than I ever thought I could be.

At the well I stuck my head under the flowing pipe and started swallowing water. I drank and drank. Then I sat down and rested a minute before I got up and drank some more. Suddenly my stomach knotted up in a terrible cramp. Then other muscles started to cramp up, in my arms and legs and back. I was wobbling on my feet when out of nowhere my head started hammering. I wanted to throw up with the pain of it.

Now, of course, I know what was going on. When water is

ingested into the stomach, it is absorbed into the bloodstream and diffused from there through to the cells. Sodium is normally present in the blood and potassium is inside the cell, and these chemicals carry on an exchange that gets the water through the cell wall and into the cell. But in the sodium-depleted state I was in back there at the well an imbalance had been set up that caused a far more rapid absorption of water than normal. In that situation the brain cells begin to swell. The brain swelling brings on severe headache, severe cramps, and severe nausea. Physiologically it's very much like heat stroke, but it's called water intoxication.

All I knew was that I was going to die. I was stretched out on the ground, and I couldn't move. My head was swimming. Katie and Charles and Bernard were trying desperately to get me up and drag me back to the house, but I was much taller and heavier, and they weren't having much luck. Finally I managed to raise myself enough so that they could get around me and prop me up. It was only a quarter mile or so to the house, but it was a rough quarter mile. We stumbled and dragged the whole way and didn't make it back till after dark.

My children, Eric and Kevin, don't believe me when I tell them about the conditions we lived with. It's hard for them to grasp, even though they've been down there often and knew my folks well. As far as they're concerned, there's all this wonderful space. You can just stand out in the middle of the fields and see forever. They'd go down and my dad would let them drive the tractor and pet the horses. Out in the fields they could just sit on one watermelon and bust another one. They could pick blackberries and go fishing in the pond. They thought that was really the way we lived, whatever I might be saying. They saw the glory side of it.

But what they see is not what I saw. That's why in 1944 I wasn't unhappy to hear that I was going out to California. The war had all the factories humming, and Daddy had already gone out there sometime earlier to take a job in the Richmond shipyards, across the bay from San Francisco. Now that he had got established and had a place to live he was sending for Mama to join him. They had work there for her too. Since Chester was a baby, she'd be taking him with her. Katie, Charles, and Bernard were going to stay with Grandma Elnora and Grandpa Charlie Reed. But Mama needed a baby-sitter for Chester, so I was going along too.

Chapter 3

Let Down Your Bucket

Uncle Slim drove us over to Texarkana in his truck so we could catch the train—Mama, Chester, and me. We got there around nightfall, so I didn't see a lot of it. But from what I did see, Texarkana was huge, with more people and traffic and buildings than I had ever thought about. Actually the population then might have been about fifteen thousand. That made it six or seven times the size of Nashville, which was pretty much my idea of a city.

From Texarkana the train rolled through Little Rock, then headed up to St. Louis and Chicago, where we changed to the Zephyr for California. Every time we stopped more passengers piled on, many of them soldiers and sailors. In the South the cars were segregated, but once we got into the North, blacks and whites rode together. Sometimes we didn't have seats, but most often we did. I held Chester on my lap and stared out the window at the farmland. Most of it seemed familiar, just bigger, except when we got into wheat country. I took notice of that. We didn't grow wheat ourselves, and I was impressed to see all that land overflowing with something I hadn't ever seen before.

The Rockies amazed me. Snow was on the peaks, and beautiful clear rivers ran alongside the tracks, different from muddy Mine Creek back home. Crossing the mountains almost made me forget how hungry I was. The food we had packed was gone after a day or so, and we didn't have money to buy much. So I was disappointed in my desire to see what eating in the dining car might be like. Denver, Salt Lake City, and Grand Junction passed by; then Reno, with a big arched sign that said THE GREATEST LITTLE CITY IN THE WORLD. In Oakland we got off at the depot and took a boat across the bay to Richmond. It was a little frightening being on such an expanse of water. But I was already adjusting to the idea of things being so different from what I was used to.

Daddy had gotten rooms for us in a big house not far outside downtown Richmond. The owners were the Reids, a man and his wife and three children, who lived in what would have been the living room and two bedrooms. The rest of the rooms they rented out, mainly to us and other members of our family. My uncle Buh and aunt Annie had one, and Uncle Bone—Boreen—had another. Mama and Daddy lived in a third with Chester, and I slept in with the Reids' two daughters. It was kind of like a big mixed-up family with everybody congregating in the kitchen to make food and eat and talk. Not that there was much time to sit around. All the adults in that house were working, some of them day shifts, some night shifts, and everybody over-time. The shipyards and factories were going around the clock. I wasn't necessarily expecting Uncle Buh and Aunt Annie and Uncle Bone to be there, but it wasn't any great surprise that they were. California was drawing people off the farms in droves, lots of them "Arkies," like I soon found out I was.

Daddy worked at the Richmond shipyards, which was where Mama went to work too, as a welder. I had never heard of Rosie the Riveter, but that's who Mama was. They took her off the farm and trained her to be a good welder. She told me last year that she could still do spot welds if it was necessary, but seams would probably be too much for her. At some point Mama quit the shipyards and was hired on at one of the canneries. Our timing worked out better that way. At the cannery she was on night shift, which meant she got home at seven in the morning, just in time to take Chester before I had to leave for school.

School in Richmond was so crowded with kids whose parents had migrated in for jobs that it had two shifts. I went first shift, seven-thirty to twelve-thirty. I had never in my life seen a school this size. It had four stories and just seemed immense. Even Nashville didn't have any four-story buildings. Most of the kids in this school were white with some Mexicans and a few blacks. Richmond had attracted many blacks from the South, but the neighborhood where we lived was mostly white, and so was the school.

This was my first time going to school with white kids, but for some reason that didn't make too much of an impression on me. There was plenty of teasing and gibing, but most of it was aimed at all the Okie, Arkie, and Tex newcomers. "The Okie told the Arkie and the Arkie told the Tex/Let's go to California and break our necks." That kind of thing went around quite a bit, and I learned that being from Arkansas wasn't necessarily something you were proud of.

What did impress me was, first, how hectic everything was, and second, how many students there were. I didn't think about it then, but the Richmond school administrators must have been doing everything they could think of to keep from drowning. The double sessions were one measure they took. Another was the placement test they gave everyone. So many of the kids were coming from rural school districts with hugely varying standards that the officials couldn't just put students in what would be their normal grade level. Some of the teenagers from schools in the Deep South could hardly read. I'm sure that most of the kids didn't even have any school records with them. I know I didn't. You just said, "Well, at home I was in the seventh grade," or tenth grade, or whatever it was that you were in.

To cope with this, the Richmond school officials made up a test to determine what grades the new students should go into. It probably wasn't very sophisticated, just something to give them a handle on the chaos. When I took it, I was placed in eighth grade, two grades above where I should have been. That was fine with me, though I didn't take it as anything especially to brag about. I knew that I was being graded against kids from very backward places. I might have been from a backward place myself, but my teachers at home had never let me coast. If I did things easily, they'd be sure to give me something harder. The result of that was that when I got to Richmond, they skipped me up twice.

The first thing I noticed about my classes was that I could compete with the white kids. The second was that what made school in Richmond different wasn't just that most of the kids were white or that there were lots more of them than I was used to. It was that many of these kids had aspirations. Some of them were sure they were going to go to college. In fact, I was in all college preparatory courses, where most of them thought that. That made an impression. For the first time it occurred to me that there might really be something in life other than being a field hand or a maid. I liked chemistry; I liked being in the laboratory. Maybe I could become something like a laboratory technician. I didn't think much more about it than that, but the idea stuck in the back of my mind. Of all my classes, the only one that didn't go well was the a cappella choir. I thought it would be really nice to sing, but when I auditioned, the director said "I really don't think you need to be in this class, Miss Jones. You've got the only absolute monotone I have ever heard."

We stayed in Richmond for two years. Eventually we moved out of the Reids' rooming house into our own apartment, and Daddy and Mama sent for the rest of the children to join us. But it wasn't too many months after that that Daddy decided it was time to go home. It must have been right about the end of the war. The factories were still booming, and everyone was still employed. By now, though, we had had money coming in steady for some time. Mama and Daddy had saved what for them must have been a nice sum. So now Daddy wanted to get back to farming. He could buy new equipment, maybe even a tractor, and really make some money. He was a farmer at heart, and a farmer always feels that next year is the year he's going to make a million dollars.

Personally I wasn't opposed to going back either. Richmond was lots better in some ways, but in others it was harder. There were no yards or fields around our apartment house, which made it more difficult to take care of my brothers and sisters. I couldn't let them play on the street, so I had to watch them constantly. I felt I was being a herder all the time. And being in charge of them from the time school was out, I wasn't able to make many friends for myself. Returning to Schaal meant going back to my friends and cousins and aunts and uncles and to my grandparents. I wasn't sad about that at all.

The train ride back wasn't nearly as memorable as the ride there, maybe because of all the children needing attention or maybe because we were heading back to the familiar instead of out into the unknown. Our old Ollie Reed house wasn't available. It probably had just deteriorated to the point of unlivability in our two years away; it wasn't far from that even when we were living in it. Instead we moved into the Old Wes Jones place, which was about a mile closer to the church and the general store. Wes Jones was bigger, five rooms instead of three, but other than that it was pretty much the same as our old house. When it rained, you still had to put pots and buckets out in a dozen places.

When we got back, I started tenth grade at the Howard County Training School in Tollette, the next town over. Tollette had been founded right after the Civil War by a group of newly freed slave families. It was still almost all black, and the Howard County Training School was a regional school for black students from as far away as Fulton and Saratoga. They were brought in from all over, and in the morning you could see fourteen or fifteen buses unloading hundreds of students in back of the school's main building.

When you think of school buses, what probably comes to mind are the traditional orange-yellow boxy affairs. Ours weren't like that. The buses that brought students into the Howard County Training School were a strange collection of home-made vehicles, many of them flatbed trucks whose owners had built some kind of structure on them that people could sit in. These weren't the kinds of buses that would pass any safety inspection today, or most likely back then either.

George Ogden's bus was like that, and the first time I got on I had a bad feeling about it. Like some of the other owners, George had taken a truck chassis and built a long flatbed onto it. On this flatbed he had constructed a rectangular wooden box, cutting out the areas where you would ordinarily expect to find windows. Of course these openings weren't windows in the sense that they had sashes and glass panes that could be opened and closed. They were just long rectangular cutouts running the length of the box on either side. George had nailed wire screening over these openings, so children wouldn't fall out, and he had fixed on rolls of burlap that could be lowered over the openings from the outside, like window shades. Most often during the school year this sacking material was kept lowered over the windows, since that was the only way to stay partway warm. At the same time some of the sacking might be raised up, since that was the only way to get some air. In any case, rolling and unrolling were done from the outside. The students inside made do with whichever way they found it. Mostly it was dark.

Inside the box the seating was also home-built. Instead of regular seats, George had rigged up wooden benches running the length of the bus on either side with two more benches running up and down in the middle. That was what I saw the first time I got on, a whole bunch of noisy kids on benches that seemed to reach back into this black hole of the bus's interior.

Standing there, looking into that dark place, I had to choke back a panic spasm. The idea of walking back there triggered off all my fears of places that could trap you in and close you up. My mind flashed back to an incident that happened when I was about five, that was engraved on my memory and still is: the time I got stuck under the house hunting eggs.

One of our barnyard hens had gotten the idea of making a nest under our house, which was built up on blocks, so there was room to get in there underneath the floor. I knew that chicken was laying eggs there, and one day I decided it was my job to go in and get them. I crawled under near the front of the house, which was blocked up a little higher than the back since the house was built on a slight grade. There was room to get in, though not much more. Then I saw that the chicken had made its nest toward the back end, where there was less space. But I still thought I could get back there. I was intending to get those eggs.

I could only crawl on all fours a little; then I had to get down on my belly and worm my way along. The underside of the house was scraping along my back as I worked up closer to the nest. Then the space narrowed down so I couldn't get there going headfirst anymore. I had to turn around and squirm toward it sideways. That way I figured I could reach my arm out and get hold of those eggs.

But before I got close enough, the space narrowed down more, and I couldn't go any farther. Stretching my arm out as far as I could, I was still too far from the nest. Then I noticed I couldn't move backward either. Somehow I had gotten wedged. As soon as I realized I was stuck, tears started welling up. I knew that crying wasn't going to do me any good. Neither was shouting, because for some reason I had chosen to go under there when nobody was home. Everybody else was out in the fields or somewhere.

I started crying anyway. I was feeling bad and scared. I was in the middle of this crying jag when I remembered something else: snakes. I wasn't absolutely sure that snakes lived under there, but they might have. Copperheads most likely, since cottonmouths liked wetness, and the ground under me was pretty dry, though dank and with that musty snake smell. Or maybe king snakes, which weren't poisonous but were big and could probably bite you pretty good anyway. I squirmed like mad, but I couldn't seem to move. I tried to get up on all fours, an impossibility. I stuck my bottom up. No luck. By now I wasn't just crying; I was shrieking.

At some point I realized someone was talking to me. When

I calmed down enough to listen, I could tell it was Dr. Tom. Dr. Tom was really my uncle Edward, but everybody always called him Dr. Tom for some reason I never knew. Dr. Tom was telling me in this very calm voice to stop crying and listen. When I finally managed to smother back my tears, I heard him say, "Now, I want you to count, Minnie. I want you to count to ten. One, two, three. C'mon, girl, just count with me." So I started counting, though I had to stop once in a while to sob some. And he was saying, "Keep counting. Keep counting, Min. Now I'm gonna reach this hoe out to you. You got to be real straight, real straight now. You catch hold to this hoe, and I'm gonna move it forward. You catch hold to it. But you got to stay flat and hold on to this hoe. Now push a little with your feet and your arms." When I saw that hoe down toward my side I grabbed on to it and didn't let go. Then, with Dr. Tom pulling the hoe and me scrabbling with my feet, I got unwedged.

Staring into the dark back of George Ogden's bus, that's what I thought about. Later I learned to get on the bus without feeling choked. I never liked it, though. I always tried to sit near the front if I could.

I had another traumatic experience on that bus, not too long after we moved into Old Wes Jones. One day at the tail end of my last class I felt like I was sitting in something wet. I was wearing a cotton print skirt with large brightly colored flowers on it, and when I pulled it around a little, I saw blood staining through the print. I wasn't feeling anything unusual, but for some reason I had just started bleeding.

I didn't know what to do first, panic because I was obviously bleeding to death or just die of embarrassment on the spot. Then I found out I could do both at the same time. As inconspicuously as I could, I glanced at the kids around me to see if they were staring. They weren't. They didn't seem to have noticed. Then I started hitching my skirt around, to get the bloody part in front instead of in back. There was only a couple of minutes left before the bell, and I figured that if the bloody part was in front, I could hold my books over it and run out to the bus that way. It wasn't easy, hitching the skirt without drawing attention to myself. But slowly, a little at a time, I maneuvered it around, pretending I was just adjusting myself, all the while practically hyperventilating with fear about what was happening to me.

When I got out to the bus, I sat down toward the back, where it was darker, which made me feel really uncomfortable. Once I was sitting down, I hitched the skirt around again, so I'd be sitting on the blood. The whole way home my fear about being back there in the dark was fighting with my fear about what might be so terribly wrong as to make me bleed down there.

As we got near my house, I pulled the skirt around again so I could hold my books in front when I stood up. When George Ogden stopped to let me out, I flew off that bus and ran into the house without stopping to say hello to Mama. There didn't seem any point in sending her into a fit too. In my room I took the skirt and underpants off, got some clean ones, and stuffed some rags in them. I did that for the next two or three days, the whole time almost crazy with worry. But then, suddenly, it stopped just as mysteriously as it had started. I was overwhelmed with relief. Whatever it was, I had been given a reprieve.

Looking back, I cannot for the life of me figure out how I couldn't have known anything about menstruation. Yet I didn't. I know that Mama had never said anything about it, which isn't a surprise by itself. Sex was a secretive thing, not to be mentioned. Children were told that babies were brought by storks, or that they came from swallowing watermelon seeds. As youngsters we spent a lot of time trying not to swallow a watermelon seed. When I got older the only advice I was given on the subject was: "Don't do it. Don't ever let no boys get on you." Mama had said that as if she meant it, but only once in passing, and she had never come back to it. That was fine with me. All I had to remember was not to do it. I did know what "it" was. I saw it practically every day of the week. Down on the farm you watch the hogs, you watch the dogs, you watch the chickens, you see all that. I couldn't quite feature what "it" might look like with people, but I had the general idea pretty clearly.

What I didn't have was any information. Sex was something you obviously knew happened, if only by the number of children around. But it certainly wasn't something people said anything about. You never talked about it. Sexuality was not a part of the atmosphere at all. Maybe menstrual periods and related subjects were things you might talk over with your older sisters. But I didn't have any older sisters. Some of my friends were menstruating, I'm sure. But I had just gotten back from two years away and had been plopped into a classful of kids two years my senior. I knew most of them, but we weren't up to exchanging intimacies yet. So there was no news from that front either.

I did learn about menstruation later on. Mama found some of my bloody clothes and told me, "When this comes on, you got to put some rags down there, so you don't mess yourself up." Then in home economics class one day Miss Dodson gave everyone a miniature pamphlet explaining the whats and the whys. She had saved the instruction manuals for us out of Kotex boxes.

School itself tended to be lots better than those bus rides. Chemistry was good; I still liked that. And math. English too, especially oratory and poetry. I didn't try out for choir; I had learned my lesson about that in Richmond. But I did have a voice that seemed to project naturally, even if I couldn't sing. People never seemed to have any trouble hearing what I had to say. So I memorized poems for the oratory contests. Paul Laurence Dunbar's dialect poetry and Langston Hughes, the great black poet from Joplin, Missouri, and Harlem, New York. I won first prize reciting Rudyard Kipling's "If."

I didn't know it then, but apparently "If" was a favorite at Negro schools. Maya Angelou, who is my contemporary and grew up in Stamps, Arkansas, about fifty miles southeast of Schaal, also talks about having learned it by heart. When I got to college, I found out that a lot of people knew the poem. Part of it, at least, might have been written specifically for American blacks of my generation:

> *If you can trust yourself when all men doubt you,*
> *But make allowance for their doubting too;*

If you can wait and not be tired by waiting,
  Or being lied about, don't deal in lies,
Or being hated, don't give way to hating,
  And yet don't look too good, nor talk too wise.

That was pretty fair advice. Not much different from what we were getting from our teachers and parents, even if they didn't say it in verse or quite so directly.

Though I hated to, I tended to miss a lot of school. In the spring of the year Katie and I and the rest stayed out to help put in the crops. In the fall the corn and cotton needed to be picked. Chester says he never did find out what started the Civil War, and he knew the outcome only from hearsay. He was always coming into school after it started and leaving before it ended.

He jokes about it now. Then we were embarrassed. The teachers would ask me why I stayed out of school so much, and I'd tell them I just didn't feel like coming. Some of them really fussed at me about it. I thought they might have noticed that I did come whenever it rained. Actually they probably knew all about why I wasn't attending and just wanted to get a discussion going. But that wasn't something I was going to discuss. I was too ashamed.

Regardless of what might have been happening in the fields, I always showed up at school for tests. I had my books, and I studied them at home, the same way I had always done my night reading, on the floor with a lamp and the covers over my head. And pretty nearly always I did the best in the class.

The fact was I liked learning too much to be put off. I didn't just like it; I loved it. A good part of that feeling came from my family. I had heard preaching on this subject from all sides from the time I could remember. I don't think it's any accident that my mother is there in my first memory teaching me to read. Grandma Minnie was another one who was constantly at me. "You've *got* to get an education": That was her refrain, like a drumbeat. "You want to pick cotton and live in all these mosquitoes the rest of your life?" There was going to be a better day if she had anything to do with it. Some kind of better day, even if she might not have been exactly sure what that day was going to look like.

As little as he said, even my father had a high regard for education. In his own way he was remarkable. Curtis Jones got through the eighth grade even though he was the oldest of seventeen children living on the edge of subsistence. He was a prime example of the dilemma our grandparents faced, and our parents. They were always saying, "Well, I couldn't go to school. But you better go there and do the best you can." Yet in order to survive, they had to keep you out of school working in the fields. It was a two-edged sword. In their hearts they were driven to see you educated. But reality often had its own ideas.

This wasn't just us. It was all the people around us. One reason for this general reverence for learning was that none of the families in Schaal and Tollette and Bright Star was very far removed from slavery. Their great-grandparents, or grandparents, sometimes even their parents had been born at a time when they weren't allowed to go to school. They weren't permitted to know how to read. They—we—were the immediate descendants of people who had huddled up in undercover schools in churches or hidden out with a teacher in the woods so they could learn their letters. So when my father came along, he was going to get as much schooling as he possibly could, even though he was a full-time field hand from the time he could lift something or carry something else.

What our parents gave us, the church reinforced. I sometimes woke up in the morning to Mama singing "I'm so glad that troubles don't last always." That wasn't too different from what Reverend Walton was preaching to us twice a month at Tabernacle Methodist and his colleague over at Bright Star Baptist the other two Sundays. Reverend Walton's favorite theme was the eagle stirring her nest. If we could see it right, what might seem trouble and hardship to us was in reality the hand of God preparing us for that better day. Reverend Walton's sermons tended to be right out of the Old Testament. Daniel in the lion's den, King David, Joshua at the walls of Jericho—they all had their trials and tribulations, their desperation and their downfalling. But God had his eye on them, like he had his eye on the sparrow. Like he had his eye on us.

I knew those lessons. From the time I was ten I was secretary of our Sunday school. So I knew them. But you didn't have to go to Sunday school to get the meaning of Joseph's life, cast by his brothers down into a pit and sold off into slavery. Or to feel it personally when the preacher stood up there in the pulpit and told us how God told Moses to tell Pharaoh to let his people go.

Those Sundays in church weren't separate from your everyday life. They were about your everyday life, and what it meant, and where it was going. Bound for the promised land didn't mean some abstract place in heaven. It might have meant that too, but it also meant bound for some better life than we had now. No matter what might be happening to you, what they told you in those little churches was that you were somebody. You were God's child.

"There were times"—this is Chester telling me what it felt like to him—"there were times when I went to church feeling so down after a week of hard labor that I was saying, 'Oh, Lord, why did you put me in this family down on this farm?' And then the preacher would say, 'God will make a way out of no way.' And all of a sudden you say, hey, it's not where I'm coming from, it's where I'm going to." That's what I felt like too, to the word.

Between what your family was saying and what the preacher was telling you, your spiritual and psychological foundation was pretty well set. There was a plan for you with a capital *P*, and that plan was to get ahead, to do better than your grandparents and parents. This was a subject my teachers hit harder than Mama and Grandma Minnie put together. You never once heard them say, "This is a good place right where you're at. This is where you want to be." It was always: "You better study. You better get this, you hear? You want to learn this? Or you want to stay down here choppin' cotton and chasin' rabbits?"

Those teachers of ours may not have had as much math or science as some others, but they instilled in us the value of being a decent human being and the value of education. They also taught us all the way along how to make it in the white world outside Howard County. "You aren't going to make it if you're only just as good as whites," they said. "You've got to be better than whites."

Negro history was part of that same lesson. Everybody in school studied that. We talked about George Washington Carver and Booker T. Washington. We read Carter Woodson, the father of Negro history, who said that if you control a man's mind, you control his actions, that we were programmed to think about ourselves the way the white world told us, but now it was time to control our own minds for ourselves. Frederick Douglass was there, and Charles Richard Drew, the great black surgeon, and of course Sojourner Truth and Harriet Tubman. Our teachers taught us that black people were people of great courage and accomplishment, that they could raise themselves up. In a dozen ways they were giving us their version of what worked. "Don't fight the system," they were saying. "Just go out there and get an education. Prove you are better."

Those were great lessons. But I wonder if our teachers weren't fighting back tears of frustration even while they were teaching them. I remember so clearly the white district supervisor saying to Miss Dodson, our home economics teacher, "Now you be sure and train your girls to be good maids." She said that every time she came around, loud enough so that we heard it too. We might have been learning pride in our race and the virtues of working to realize a better day. But all the while we were studying home economics half a day every day for five years, seventh grade through twelfth. I laugh. I tell people, "I'm the best maid I know." And I am. I don't know of anybody who understands how to clean a house like I do, not that I want to do it. Or prepare a meal. We had to be well trained so that when we would come to your home, we would know how to clean it, know where things ought to be, know how to set your table, know how to do it right. We couldn't do it in our own houses, but we sure did know how it was done.

I might have been trained for maid work, but I don't know

that I ever actually thought I would be doing it. The fact was that I didn't have the slightest notion what I would do. That lab technician idea was still hovering around somewhere, though how I might ever become one wasn't very clear. What I did know was that I had no interest in being like any of the women I knew. None of them struck me as someone I wanted to emulate.

Looking at my mother and grandmother, I certainly didn't want to be like them. Later on I was able to see their lives as farm women and mothers for the successes they were. There's no question that all the children in our family were secure and all of us felt loved. But at the time I took those things for granted. Anybody who wanted to could have children, so that didn't seem like all that much of an accomplishment. I was an adult before I realized how wonderful it was to have seven sisters and brothers. Back then I would have liked to have had none. I didn't have any I particularly wanted to get rid of, but neither did I see it as a great honor to have a big family.

If I had to characterize the women I grew up around, I would say that most of them were submissive. They tried to please their husbands. They worked very hard and got very little. And they were always striving with all their might to take care of their children. I must have heard my mother say a thousand times, "Lord, just let me live to raise my last child. That's all I ask."

But many of them also harbored the idea that as soon as the children were grown, they were going to make tracks out of there. I heard my mother say that often too, but I'm not just talking about my mother. None of them ever did it, though. As soon as their children actually were grown, we didn't hear that anymore. If you talked to Mama in her later years, she'd say, "Well, I got to take care of your daddy." But thirty plus years ago it was that they were going to get out. I think that was the pressures and frustrations of their lives speaking, that and their unhappy feelings about being so dependent on their men.

Those men. Characterize them, and you're talking about work, grinding, energy-sapping, always-more-to-do physical work. That's one. Two is that none of them ever did a stitch of housework. If we hadn't eaten in the kitchen, my father wouldn't have known where it was. They didn't cook or clean or take care of a baby or change a diaper. I don't ever remember seeing a man do that until I saw my husband, Oliver, changing our boys. Those men loved their families, and they took their responsibilities to heart. But as I grew up, I never felt that any of them were as respectful of their wives as they should have been. Who pleased and who got pleased was pretty much a one-way street.

My view on this subject might have gotten jaundiced from the one time my father ever hit my mother, which I saw. I couldn't have been very old when this happened, but I was old enough to remember what it looked like and why it happened. Mama had been trying to burn out a nest of mites in the chicken house, but something must have gotten away from her, and the whole thing caught fire.

Daddy was fussin' at her about what she had done, it was so stupid. And she was saying something about it, probably trying to explain herself in some way. But he was really hot, and the chicken house wasn't all that far from the main house, which maybe could have gone up as well. And in his frustration he hit her. It took me a long, long time to let go of my anger at him for that. I'm talking about many years. It probably wouldn't have bothered me nearly so much if that kind of thing had been common. But it didn't happen much in Schaal. In our families somebody beating his wife would have shocked and appalled the whole clan. I also remembered very well that Daddy said he had promised himself he would never hit his family. So that made me doubly mad.

From that moment on I was just absolutely determined that no man was ever going to hit me. Long after Oliver and I were married we had a neighbor who used to beat his wife. One day he came over and we got into a big argument about something. In the heat of the moment he drew back his fist as if he were going to punch me. When I saw that, I picked up the biggest thing that was handy, which happened to be a large potted plant, and heaved it at him. It missed him but smashed through a big window with a crash and glass shards all over the place. That kind of snapped him out of it. "Now, Joycelyn," he said, "you know I wasn't going to hit you."

I said, "I *know* you weren't!"

Since then my two boys say, "You try to do anything to Mama, and she goes crazy."

———

Though I didn't think Mama and Grandma and the rest got the respect they deserved, I personally didn't feel put upon in some way because I was a girl. I never heard anybody say that being a girl, I couldn't do as well as boys. I also wasn't bothered by being younger than my classmates. It wasn't something I particularly noticed, and I think they probably didn't either. I had taken care of a lot of children by then and run a lot of farmwork, so my exact chronology didn't make much difference. On top of that, I had done well. I was at the top of my class, which admittedly wasn't saying all that much since by twelfth grade there were only nine of us left. Almost everybody at Howard County Training got up to the eighth or ninth grade. But then they started dropping like flies, the boys off to the farm, the girls off to marry the boys. By senior year the attrition rate must have been 90 percent.

High school graduation was probably the biggest black event of the year in Howard County, regardless of how small the class might be. The auditorium held about five hundred, and there wouldn't be room to squeeze everybody inside. Graduations were entertainment, something to do and people to see. But they were also emotional, important occasions. So few of the students who started out actually finished that those who did seemed precious in the eyes of those who watched. I may not have actually been the first in my family to finish high school. I think one or two of my aunts and uncles may have done it before me. But it was unusual enough to be something special. Mama and Grandma Minnie had had their hearts set on this moment for years.

The first part of graduation was what was called Baccalaureate. This was a kind of presenting the graduates to the community ceremony that was always held on the Sunday before commencement. We all marched in shining with pride in our white caps and gowns. Under my gown I was wearing the prettiest dress I had ever seen, or at least the prettiest I had ever owned, made of a white, silky material with a white-on-white stripe in it and a tie belt around the waist. Homemade, of course, by Miss Beatrice, who did everybody's fine work in Schaal. The nine of us were introduced. Then we sat there facing the packed school auditorium while a preacher gave the invocation and preached, and another speaker made a speech.

Sitting there in front of that crowd, I was too taken up with the whole thing to listen that intently to what they were saying. At least I can't remember any of it now. The fact is I can barely remember the valedictorian speech I gave the following Thursday night at the diploma ceremony. I do remember the title of that, though. It was "Let Down Your Bucket Where You Are." I got that from one time at Grandma Minnie's when she had sent me out to draw a bucket of water and I had taken too much time doing it for her liking. What happened was that the area around the well was muddy from a rainstorm and I had a hard time finding a good place to stand so I could lower the bucket. When I didn't get back fast enough, Grandma Min yelled out, "What's going on down there?" And when I shouted back that I was trying to find a place to stand, she said, "Just let down your bucket where you are." That struck me as good advice generally, and still does. The speech I made from it was about doing the absolute best you can wherever you find yourself and whatever the circumstances.

I think I don't remember the actual speech because I was too nervous in front of that auditorium. Pride and nerves are about all I do remember from that commencement. Except that all of us were wondering about the white man who was sitting up on the stage with Mr. Turner, the school principal. None of us had any idea of who he was until he got up and made a short announcement. He was a professor, he said, representing Philander

Smith College in Little Rock and the United Methodists. Philander Smith was a fine Methodist college, and he was there to award a full-tuition scholarship to the class valedictorian. He didn't mention me by name, but I had just given the speech. So it was pretty clear that I was the one he was talking about.

Chapter 4

Do We Have Enough Yet?

❧

This surprise scholarship news didn't make as big an impact as it might have. That was because from where I was standing that summer it didn't look like I would actually get to go anywhere. July was when we chopped cotton and corn, which meant I was out in the fields like always, which was where Daddy needed me to be. Of course Mama wanted desperately for me to go, and I knew they were bickering about it. But college had never been part of their world, so the idea of it seemed strange and unusual. What going to college might mean for the future wasn't that obvious to Daddy. But he could see clear as day that if I went off, he'd be losing his work leader. If it was between him and Mama, I knew that when September rolled around, I wouldn't be anywhere near Little Rock. I'd be picking cotton.

Peach season came at the end of July. By then the chopping was more or less done, and we were free to hire ourselves out to the peach orchards. Everyone liked that, for two reasons. On your own farm you worked day in, day out with your own set. But picking peaches, you had a chance to get away from family and socialize. You could also earn some hard money. Forty cents an hour for a ten-hour day was a serious contribution to your cash flow. Peach picking was the best job around.

The way it worked was that the orchard owners would con-
tract with a man who owned a truck. The trucker would be
responsible for hiring and paying the hands, getting them to the
job, and harvesting the fruit. If he signed you on, he'd come by
your house every morning to get you. By the time he made the
rounds his flatbed would be full up with young people from the
neighborhood. We'd spend all day together picking peaches,
then be gathered up again at sundown for the ride back. My
uncle Slim was a trucker, in addition to his dairy farming and
bootlegging. He ran his truck all through the summer, making
contracts for the early crop in July, then a second crop in August,
when more pickers were available.

By the time August came to an end I wasn't thinking about
college anymore. The cotton crop would be ready for a first
picking in September, right about when Philander Smith was
supposed to start. That was our real cash crop, and Daddy
would need every hand. I knew he had beat Mama down on
the issue, despite how badly she wanted me to go. So that was
that. I had no hint whatsoever that a higher authority was about
to intervene. But it did, suddenly and unexpectedly, in the person of Grandma Minnie.

Grandma Minnie of course, right alongside Mama, had kept
up the drumbeat for years about me going to school. Now, a
week or so before the beginning of the semester, she put her
foot down. She might have been waiting to see if Daddy was
going to relent and let me go. Or maybe it had just taken her
that long to make up her own mind. Whichever, early in September she decided it was time to have her say. I heard about
it almost offhand. One day, apropos of nothing, she just told
me, "All right, honey, now you go ahead on up there. I've got
enough shoulders around here for you to stand on." Daddy
might have been a stern authoritarian, but when his mama made
a pronouncement like that, there was no more talking to be
done. That was all the consideration required.

After that the only problem was money. The end of August,
beginning of September was always a hard time. I can't say for
sure what our cash income might have been in any given year,

but I'd be surprised if it was much more than five hundred dollars. Some came from the coonskins and some from peach picking and then the bulk from cotton. Out of that we had to buy sugar, coffee, and flour. Those were essential. Also shoes and cloth and tools and seed and coal oil and supplemental food for the animals, like those shorts we fed the hogs with, and no doubt some other things that I'm forgetting.

The overall result was that we seldom had more than a few dollars around the house, and often not that. Mama remembered picking and selling blackberries to buy a set of diapers when I was born. Before Christmas she sometimes went out coon hunting with Daddy so she'd have money for presents. Not long ago Oliver and I were looking through some old family papers, and we came across a sixty-year-old mortgage document on pigs. Daddy had taken out a loan against seven of his hogs to tide him over some especially lean time. Anyway, the end of August was hard. By then the peach money was already gone. The coonskin money was back in the winter months, and the cotton money would come only with the fall harvest. When we asked up at the high school, we were told that the Methodist scholarship paid for the tuition and that Philander Smith would arrange some kind of part-time job for me that would take care of my room and board. That left the bus fare up to Little Rock, $3.83. Which we didn't have.

Ordinarily we didn't start picking cotton until a little later in September. There was often some early cotton to be had a few weeks before that, but it wasn't usually worth bothering about. You'd just wait until the crop was ready for a major picking. But that year the whole family got out into the cotton patch, scouring for whatever bolls might have ripened early. My main recollection of that is how tired we were, but one image is carved on my memory. It was toward nightfall one day when Chester looked up at me from where he was stooped over. He was five years old, and he had been working since sunup. "Min," he asked, "do we have enough yet?"

We sold that cotton for five dollars, I think to Fred Jones, one of Old Man Will Jones's boys. Will Jones had three children:

Wes, whose old house we were living in; May, who had married Ray Dorsey; and Fred, who lived up the road from May. Fred was probably doing the best of all of them at that time, so the chances are that he was the one who bought our cotton. Which gave us the money for a bus ticket, with a dollar and change left to spare.

When the day came, Mama and I packed my clothes in an old suitcase, and I put on my traveling outfit, a plaid dress with a white collar that Miss Beatrice had made and my black-and-white saddle oxfords and bobby socks. I thought I looked about as smart as I could look. I didn't know that bobby socks weren't allowed at Philander Smith College. They held a strictly conservative view on life up there that frowned on women's socks as being overly sporting. Philander Smith required women to wear stockings when they went to class and whenever they went off campus. Of course I didn't know any of this at the time, fortunately, since I don't know where I would have gotten stockings from.

With all the last-minute excitement, I was already waiting for Uncle Slim to come get us in his truck before I realized how confused I was about going. I wanted to go, that was for sure. I had been thinking about college since my high school in Richmond. But to be actually standing there with my suitcase waiting for Uncle Slim to take me to the bus, that was a completely different thing from just thinking about it. For the first time it hit me that I was really leaving. Except for California, I had spent my entire just-turned sixteen-year-old life in the bosom of my family and friends. Even in Richmond Mama and Daddy were there, and Uncle Buh and those, and Chester, and then the rest. Of course there was nothing in Schaal to look forward to except more field work, but at least down here I knew everybody. It might have been hard, but it was a comfortable hard.

Maybe that was why I had a queasy feeling sitting on the bed of Uncle Slim's truck between my suitcase and Charles, who had come for the ride to the bus station in Mineral Springs. Mama and Grandma Elnora were squeezed up front in the cab with Uncle Slim. Mama and Charles were just along to say good-bye, but Grandma Elnora had decided to keep me company all the way to Little Rock, to make sure I got there all right.

In Mineral Springs we bought our tickets at the drugstore, then we stood out on the little platform in front to wait for the bus. When it finally came, I hugged Mama good-bye and gave Charles a squeeze. Then Grandma Elnora and I got on and walked to the back of the bus. Neither of us gave a second's thought to where we sat down. Rosa Parks wasn't going to come along for another six years.

When we got up to Little Rock, it was a day or two before classes were supposed to start. Grandma Elnora delivered me to the house of one of her cousins who lived in North Little Rock; then after a bit we said good-bye, and she went back to the bus station. The next day the cousin's daughter took me by bus to Philander Smith—my first sight of an actual college.

Philander Smith was founded by former slaves not long after the Civil War and was one of the country's oldest black colleges. But I didn't know any of that. I had no idea what to expect. The first thing I saw was a crowd of students gathered around one of the buildings, so I went over there and found out that was the place to register. The first line I got in went up to a desk where you settled on your classes. That wasn't hard because if you were a freshman or sophomore, they more or less told you what you had to study. Then I went over to another desk where there was an adviser who had to sign off and approve what I was taking. When that was done, I got in another line that led into the business office, where you were meant to pay your bills.

Standing in this line, I began to get nervous. Everyone seemed to be talking about money for tuition, but they all sounded like they knew what to expect, and they all seemed to have everything in order. The only thing I knew was that I was supposed to have a scholarship. The white professor had announced it at commencement, and I had been told by the high school office. But nobody had given me any papers or sent a letter or anything

I could show to the person at the counter who was checking people off. The only thing I had with me was me.

When my turn came, the lady at the counter looked at my class cards and told me I owed eight hundred dollars. I tried to explain about my scholarship and my job, but I couldn't seem to make any headway. Minnie Lee Jones wasn't a name on her list. There was no indication of my scholarship, or of where I was meant to stay, or of any job I was supposed to have to earn my board and keep. "I'm sorry," the woman said, "we have no record of you at all. If you want to register, the tuition is eight hundred dollars."

When I heard what she was saying, I got frightened. It wasn't that I started seeing visions of cotton rows, but I had no idea what to do about this, and the mention of a sum like eight hundred dollars made me so upset I began to feel dizzy. With a whole line of people still waiting, the accounts lady said I should probably go over to the president's office and talk to them. I wandered off slowly into the hallway in a kind of daze, without the least notion what to do. I don't think the idea of seeing the president really registered. This didn't look like the kind of thing that I was going to be able to work out. Somehow they had forgotten they gave me a scholarship. Or maybe there was something we were supposed to have done that we just hadn't understood right. Whatever had happened, according to Philander Smith College, I wasn't a student.

I was standing there in the hall, feeling lost and forlorn, when a voice said to me, "Young lady, what seems to be the matter? What kind of trouble are you having?" The voice that said this was not the sort you heard every day of the week. It was a deep, dark voice, a little nasal, but kind, with no touch of harshness to it. The words came in a slow country drawl. They sounded like they were emerging out of some cavern in the depths of the earth.

When I looked up, I saw the most enormous human being I had ever seen in my life. A giant black man was looking down at me. My first thought was not to try to estimate his measurements; it was just a kind of shock at how a person could grow so immense. Now, after being married all these years to Oliver, who was a famous basketball coach in Arkansas before he retired, I would do an instant take on the man's height, which was probably six feet ten or eleven. He was not fat, but he was heavily built and well proportioned, like Shaquille O'Neal except a shade shorter, but with a mature man's thickness. He was a tower. His name, he said, was Reverend M. Lafayette Harris, and he was the president of Philander Smith College.

I took a deep breath, and then the words came tumbling out. I told him that I was from Schaal and that I thought I had a scholarship and they were going to get me a job, but now nobody could find any record of me. And he said, "Well, young lady, let me see what I can do to take care of you." Then he moved off into the office I had just come out of. When he came back a minute later, he drawled, "You just go on down to Adeline Smith Hall. You go down there and tell them I said to get you a place to sleep tonight. Tomorrow I'll find something for you to do."

As it turned out, my name was not on the registrar's list of enrollees who had gone through the normal application process. Instead it was on a separate list of high school valedictorians who had been awarded scholarships, which was a method Philander Smith had started using to recruit people they thought would be good students. I had never formally applied to the college or requested a dorm or done anything; that was why the registrar had never heard of me.

I might have thought it was pure luck, meeting the college president in the hallway. But actually there was nothing so unusual about it, as I learned after I had been there awhile. Philander Smith was M. Lafayette Harris's personal preserve. He dominated the school with his presence. Everyone had a story about him, and the last thing anybody wanted to do was get on his wrong side. He seemed to be a serene man mostly, but what he might be capable of doing if he ever did get mad was the subject of considerable curiosity and speculation.

I've since seen small colleges where the president's wife ends up being a mother hen to everybody and the president himself is a kind of recluse. But at Philander Smith Mrs. Harris was not so much the mother hen as Reverend Harris was the father on high, which was what some of the students called him. The Harrises lived right on campus, and the president himself was everywhere all the time. Every student saw M. Lafayette Harris every day. This was his place. He was president for thirty years or so and left only when he was appointed bishop of Kansas City. The Reverend Lafayette Harris was an institution all by himself.

My roommate that first year was Joyce Montgomery, who was Oliver's first cousin, though I wasn't to meet Oliver himself for another ten years. Joyce was eighteen or nineteen, maybe three years older than I was and just as happy and friendly as could be. She was and still is a completely delightful person. Joyce had come up from the little town of Almyra, Arkansas, on a basketball scholarship. Philander Smith didn't have much of a football team, but they were good at basketball, both men's and women's, and Joyce was a real player as well as a good student.

Not everybody there was from a small town. I met girls from Little Rock, and there were many from Ohio—Cincinnati, Columbus, and Cleveland—girls who seemed extremely sophisticated. One, who was from Arkansas, was exceptionally prim and proper. She acted as if she had been raised in a wealthy upper-crust family, though we were sure she must have come from the same kind of background the rest of us did. She'd ask, "Shall we have tea now?" which would make everyone smile. If I had ever said such a thing, they would have fallen down laughing.

Of all the new students, Joyce was one of the most popular. She was tall and pretty and intelligent, and right from the start she took me under her wing, so things began to fall into place socially. Very soon I had a job too, scrubbing floors in the bathrooms and hallways in the girls' dorm. That didn't seem so terrible at all. I did have to be on my hands and knees some, but it was lots better than picking cotton. Joyce's expenses were paid by her basketball scholarship, but most of the girls had some kind of job, whether it was in the laundry or kitchen or cleaning, like I was doing. Practically everything at Philander Smith that needed doing was done by students working to pay part of their bills.

I don't recall there being any particular orientation before classes started. That doesn't mean there wasn't one, just that I don't remember it. I do have a very distinct memory, though, of a day or two spent rushing around in confusion, looking for where classes were supposed to be, which is what all the freshmen were doing. Another thing that sticks in my mind is the freshman physical exam, when two or three hundred of us lined up at the infirmary to have our chests listened to, our blood pressures taken, and our teeth looked at. What made that event memorable was that it was the first time I had ever personally seen a doctor. At Bright Star and Howard County Training I had been examined by public health nurses. They gave us eye tests, looked for clubfeet, and administered smallpox vaccinations. But this was my first visit to an actual doctor. Other than Bernard when his appendix burst, no one in our family had ever been to see one.

My first class was freshman English with Dr. Pipes, who now teaches at Michigan State. He was another large man, though not so enormous as Reverend Harris, and very bright. He pushed us hard to learn grammar and to write decently. Dr. Pipes graded on content and style, and the first story I wrote for him got an A over F, A for content. I found out soon that my high school English training was not all it might have been. Of course that was true for a lot of other girls too, especially the ones from rural areas. But Dr. Pipes knew what he was dealing with. He was experienced and inventive, and the learning curve in his class was pretty steep.

I took algebra, which wasn't bad, and biology and chemistry and German. You needed to have a foreign language, and I was told that German was the right one to know if you were going to study science. Even now I can read German decently. I can't necessarily sit down and pronounce it so that a German speaker would understand anything, but I can still read a scientific article well enough to know what the conclusion is.

I also found out what language it was that Red Schaals had been speaking back home. Schaal was named after a white family that was still there when I was growing up, and Red Schaals, one of their sons, was about my age. They owned land and lots of cattle, but what was strange was how they spoke differently in their house. We couldn't understand them at all. No one identified it as German, just that it was some incomprehensible manner of speaking. Among other things, my German class cleared up that little mystery.

From the start I did fairly well in my courses, well enough so that it looked like I'd make dean's list, for which you needed a B average as a freshman. That didn't surprise me particularly. It hadn't occurred to me that anything else might be possible. After all, I had gotten good grades out in California, and I had been first at Howard County Training School. I guess what did surprise me was that I wasn't doing even better. In fact that bothered me quite a lot at first. But I didn't have much time to worry about it. I was studying hard and working a lot to pay off my bills, and the months just seemed to fly by.

I couldn't afford to go home for Thanksgiving, but before the Christmas vacation Mama sent me money for a bus ticket. I was really excited about seeing my brothers and sisters again. I wanted to tell them about everything I was doing. Looking back on it, I can see that this was probably an even bigger event for them than it was for me. Before I ended up going, the idea of college was too exotic and distant for them even to think about. But now "college" had gotten into their vocabulary. And here I was, coming back with news from beyond.

On the bus ride from Little Rock I was thinking more and more that I should be bringing some kind of present with me. I wanted to have something for Katie and Charles and Bernard and the rest. I had actually been thinking about this since I knew I was going home. But my total money supply was thirty-seven cents that I think must have been left over from the ticket money Mama had sent. So I hadn't been able to get anything, which was bothering me considerably.

The bus went from Little Rock to Hot Springs, where I was supposed to change for Mineral Springs. Waiting at the bus station in Hot Springs, I looked around, and there behind the candy counter was a big box of bite-size Baby Ruth candy bars. That looked like just the thing. When I asked, the man said the Baby Ruths were forty cents, which left me three cents shy. I felt a wave of sadness and depression. It just seemed right that as the oldest I should bring back a present. But there was no way to do it. Just as I was despairing over this, the white lady standing next to me caught my eye. She had also ridden on the bus to Hot Springs and was waiting for a connection. She had seen what happened. "Well," she said, "I've got three pennies. Why don't you go ahead and get it?"

When Uncle Slim delivered me home from the bus stop in Mineral Springs, all the kids came spilling out of the house hollering. Mama gave me a big warm hug, and Daddy stood there smiling. "Well, Mint," he said, "we're glad to have you back." I didn't make Katie and the rest wait till Christmas either. They were really excited about those little Baby Ruth pieces, and they were all hovering around me, laughing and talking. I felt like a mother hen with chicks. And when I started telling them about college, they hung on every word. I was their big sister, and I was going to college, and as soon as they got big enough, they all were going to go to college too.

The next morning we went out into the woods to cut a Christmas tree, same as always. Then we got out the old decorations, some Christmas tree balls and the silver rope that we draped around the tree and the tinsel. Mama killed a chicken for our traditional baked chicken and dressing Christmas dinner, and we also baked a raccoon with different kinds of vegetables. And pies, lots of pies—sweet potato, lemon, chocolate and a cake and cookies. That was what Christmas was about at our house.

Everyone went to bed early Christmas Eve so you could get up first thing next morning and open your gifts and start eating more cake. Then we went off to church for services to hear Reverend Walton's sermon on the birth of the baby Jesus. There I had been away in a different world entirely for three and a half months, and now I came back to find things exactly the way I thought they would be.

I was just so glad to be home and to be with my sisters and brothers. We went fishing together, and we went to see all my aunts and uncles, always eating everywhere we went. Mama was constantly telling me, "Now you got to go see this person, you got to go see that person." If there was someone in Schaal I didn't visit that Christmas, it wasn't for lack of trying.

Between visiting I just seemed to slip back into the flow of the house. I chopped lots of wood, hauled water, pulled peanuts, hulled peas, and shucked corn. At night I slept with my sister Katie, just as I always had. I was happy as a clam.

———

At Philander Smith one of the things I had heard about first semester was the sororities: the Deltas, AKAs, Zetas, and Sigma Gamma Rhos. They and their male counterparts, the Kappas, Alphas, Omegas, and Sigmas, more or less dominated student life. Almost all the student leaders seemed to be members of one or another. These weren't the kinds of sororities most people think of, where the main purpose is to get dates and have parties. Delta, AKA, and the others were national organizations of professional women who kept their numbers growing by recruiting college students. I didn't know it at the time, but these sororities were part of the black world's answer to being excluded from the elite groups of the white establishment. They and similar black brotherhoods and sisterhoods represented accomplishment and status in a society that had no interest in recognizing black achievement. So their importance went far beyond that of the usual college fraternities. Of course I wasn't aware of this back then or maybe only in the vaguest way imaginable. All I really knew about the sororities was that joining one was a prestigious thing to do and that being asked was an honor. Then at the beginning of the second semester I started getting visits from the most unusual, high-powered group of black women I had ever encountered.

It was a little overwhelming and really very flattering to realize I was being courted by all four sororities. A few months earlier I had never heard of any of them. But by now I knew that you just had to be a member of one if you wanted to be anyone. Joyce Montgomery was joining the AKAs, who seemed wonderful. But I was even more impressed by the Delta Sigma Theta women who were coming around to talk. These weren't students; they were adult women, some from the outside world and some from the Philander Smith faculty. One of them was Sue Cowan Williams, who was an official in the state department of education and was well known as a pioneering black professional. Another was Forrestine Williams, who was head of the board of black cosmetology in Arkansas and whose daughter Florine was a good friend and classmate of mine. Others were business people or administrators or educators. These were women I admired and respected tremendously, and still do. They were in the kinds of positions I didn't know that women could have. I understood they were doing important things.

What they talked about mostly was how they had gotten to where they were and what it meant to them and what it meant to them to be a Delta. If you were chosen, you became a part of the Delta sisterhood. You had a real responsibility to your sisters and to all young black women, for whom you would be a role model. You had an obligation to achieve and make the most of your potential, and you could never do anything that would embarrass the name of Delta. I thought these were serious, impressive people. They gave me the idea that I might become like them someday. What they were saying seemed so right.

In the end Florine Williams and I and seven other girls became Pyramids, which is what the Delta pledges were called. On certain days of the week we had to wear something red and something white, which were the Delta colors, and we had to study together and eat together. We also had to do public service work, at the college since freshmen were rarely allowed off campus. I was exceptionally proud and happy to be a Pyramid.

Each Sunday the student body at Philander Smith had to attend church service. Then on Wednesdays we had mandatory "chapel" in Bud Long Hall, where Dr. Harris would speak to us. Once a month or so there'd be a chapel where the program was planned by one of the college organizations, often a sorority or fraternity. The one Delta was in charge of they gave over to the Pyramids.

After some talk we decided we wanted to invite Edith Irby to come and speak. Edith Irby, who later became Edith Irby Jones, was a Delta. She was also a medical student at the University of Arkansas, but not just an ordinary medical student. Edith Irby was the first black medical student and also one of the first women medical students. At the university medical school she was scaling two barriers at once. Of course Delta was very proud of her, but it wasn't just Delta. Everybody was proud of her. Edith Irby cut a high profile in Arkansas's black community.

Nowadays when I talk about Edith Irby Jones and what she meant to all of us, and especially to me personally, she shrugs it off. She tells people, "Oh, she's just saying that. I never did a thing for her." She says that, but at some level I think she's aware of the impact her life made on others. She later became a well-known internist and professor of medicine at Baylor and then at the University of Texas. Along the way she picked up dozens of honors and served for a time as president of the National Medical Association. Edith Irby blazed trails.

Although Edith was the first black student in the medical school, she wasn't the first black student at the University of Arkansas. In fact Arkansas was the first state university in the old South to be integrated. It started in 1948, very slowly and without fanfare, fifteen years before George Wallace plumped himself down in the doorway at the University of Alabama and fourteen years before James Meredith won admission in Mississippi. Instead of opening the whole university up at once, Arkansas did it in stages, beginning with the professional schools.

First came the law school, which in the spring of 1948 admitted Silas Hunt, from Texarkana. From our viewpoint now, more than a half century later, starting with the professional schools seems like it might have been a humane and civilized approach to integration. But Silas Hunt's stay wasn't gracious. He had been admitted, but he was isolated in a separate study room in the basement of the law building. In class they built a kind of boarded area to keep him apart from the others. Many white students accepted him, but others assaulted him with obscenities and filth.

Unfortunately Silas Hunt never graduated from the law school. In the summer after his enrollment he became so ill he had to withdraw. Less than a year later he died of tuberculosis, complicated by wounds he had suffered in World War II at the Battle of the Bulge. It's impossible to say what might have come of him or how time would have affected his feelings. I never met Silas Hunt, and I don't know how he thought about the indignities he met with. Perhaps he would have been like Hamilton Holmes, who along with Charlayne Hunter (now Hunter-Gault) broke the color barrier at the University of Georgia. Hamilton Holmes was bitter about the racist mobs and attacks he endured. But later in his life as a prominent physician he became the University of Georgia's first black trustee and endowed scholarships there for black students. He said at one point that improving the university would "benefit everyone in Georgia, blacks and whites." Maybe Silas Hunt would have said something similar in the due course of time; I don't know. But I do know that just last year the University of Arkansas's main campus in Fayetteville named its new admissions and financial aid building after him.

So Silas Hunt integrated the law school and Edith Irby did the same for the medical school. I was in charge of our Pyramids' program committee, but I didn't personally talk to her about coming to speak. So I had never actually seen Edith Irby before the Wednesday she gave her talk. I was sitting there in Bud Long Hall with everyone else when this beautiful, petite woman walked in wearing a white suit that set off her rich brown skin. She had a roundish face and a big smile, and when she started speaking, a kind of husky voice came out that sounded like it belonged to someone larger and more robust.

Her talk was about the high road and the low, and how some people rest content with the low road, or the middle ground, instead of striving for the heights. She used a poem that brought it all together. "Some of us take the high road/Others take the low/And in between on misty paths/The rest walk to and fro."

Once Edith Irby started to speak I couldn't take my eyes off her. I was captivated. I thought I had never seen anyone as beautiful or heard anything as moving. I didn't know about anybody else in that hall, but as for me, I knew what I was going to do. I was going to take the high road. All I could think of was that I wanted to be exactly like her and do exactly what she was doing.

Chapter 5

The Only One

❧❧❧

Up at the law school in Fayetteville, Silas Hunt's life was rough. But Edith Irby Jones says the medical school wasn't like that at all. She went in with young men who were five or six years older than she was, many of whom had served in World War II. They had come back from the service to finish college, and they needed to get on with their lives. They didn't have time to bother with foolishness about whom they might be sitting next to. "They formed a protective shield around me," she says.

I didn't know anything about that. Neither did I know that the way Edith got the money for medical school was that her neighbors in Hot Springs raised five hundred dollars by passing their hats. Even with that she was still forty dollars short when she got to Little Rock, so she went to Daisy Bates, one of the matriarchs of Little Rock's black community. Daisy Bates and her husband, L.C., ran the *Arkansas State Press,* the major black newspaper. When she was faced by this young girl she had never seen before who needed forty dollars to enroll, she went right to her cashbox and got out the money. Edith says she found out years later that the money Daisy Bates gave her was the entire cash supply the *State Press* had in its possession. I wish I had known those things; they would have given me even better hope.

But actually, listening to her that day was all the inspiration I needed. It was as if in that whole crowded auditorium she had been sending out her words right specifically from her lips to my ears.

After hearing Edith Irby, I felt a sense of purpose that was completely new to me. Before that I only had this vague idea it would be nice to work in a lab. So that's what I had been shooting for. Now I knew with 100 percent certainty that I was going to go to medical school and become a doctor.

Of course I didn't know yet how I was going to do it. My parents weren't going to have the money to send me, that was for sure. Still, I was certain I could find a way. Maybe it was the optimism of youth, but I was convinced that if I worked hard enough and looked hard enough, somehow I'd get there.

The next time I went home was late that spring. At Philander Smith there was no spring break like most schools had. We celebrated Easter right there and worked straight through. That way they could let us out in early May, so students could find jobs or get into the fields in time for cultivating or late planting.

When I arrived back in Schaal, cotton chopping had already started. That evening I unpacked my suitcase and helped cook dinner. Early next morning I got up, put on an old work dress, long cotton stockings, and a head scarf, and went out to the fields with Mama and Daddy and the rest. Out there, working in the cotton rows, I got my first indication that college was beginning to make a change in me.

The day was hot. Early on the sun began to blaze. The whole crew was chopping hard, and so was I. But after a while my hands began to hurt. My palms were getting rubbed raw. I hid it and kept the pace up. But the work was starting to wear me out. As the day went on, I felt I might have to quit and sit down. I would have too, except I couldn't bring myself to do it in front of my sisters and brothers. They were used to me being the work leader, not someone who quit before quitting time. There was no way I was going to let down, even if I had to end up dropping dead. Besides, I couldn't understand what my problem was. I had only been chopping cotton all my life, in hotter weather than this too.

It took me awhile to realize that if you're working all winter and spring, you can ease into chopping without its being any kind of special strain. You just move right along from spring work into summer. But you can't go straight from sitting in a classroom for eight or nine months to full speed ahead chopping. At least I couldn't. As the day stretched on, I fought it out. I just wasn't going to let the rest of them down or have them think I was slacking. I don't remember how I made it through until dinner. But somehow I did, even if at the end of work my palms looked like an advertisement for blisters.

That should have told me that at least in some ways I wasn't exactly the same person I had been when I left. Not that I actually did see it that way. I just thought I was a little out of practice as far as chopping cotton went. But there were some other signs of change too. Watching my mother bent over a grubbing hoe all day, I caught myself feeling sorry for her, the first time in my life that thought ever dawned on me. Along with it the idea came to me that I'd better hurry up and finish college so I could get a real job and help her and the others out.

Of course I grew up knowing how hard Mama worked. I had understood for a long time that whatever I might do, I did not want to lead the same kind of life she and the other women down there did. But being sorry for her was something completely different. The first time I ever had that feeling was right then when I got back from college. But every time I came back afterward it hit me harder. I did not want her to have to live like that. I didn't know anything I could do about it except get out and work to help her out, which was a drive that motivated me for a long time afterward. Not that anybody was ever going to change her life, not back then and especially not later. But thinking back on it, I realize that feeling like that meant I was beginning to look at the person I was differently from the way I had seen myself before. A year in college wasn't going to separate me from my roots. Nothing could do that, ever. But it had started me thinking about where I came from in relation to wherever it was I might be heading.

I didn't stay in Schaal long. I was there for a brief time. Then I went to Kansas City, where my aunt Joella and uncle Tommy had arranged a job for me. Aunt Jo was one of Daddy's sisters. She and Uncle Tommy had moved to Kansas City, where she owned a beauty parlor and he worked at a meat-packing company. They had a nice brick house on a hill with four bedrooms and always loved having visitors. I was the first one of Curtis and Haller's children to stay with them, but later on many of my brothers and sisters did too for different lengths of time. To some of us Aunt Jo and Uncle Tommy got to be like second parents.

My job that summer was as a live-in maid, so I didn't have much free time. But I did get Sundays off, and every Sunday I went with Aunt Jo and Uncle Tommy to watch the Kansas City Monarchs play baseball at the park they shared with the Blues, the white minor-league team. The Monarchs were maybe the most famous team in the Negro Leagues. Cool Papa Bell, one of the greatest ballplayers ever, played for them at that time. So did Satchel Paige and Buck O'Neil, who both went to the Baseball Hall of Fame, and Frank Duncan, the catcher, who lived just a couple of doors from Aunt Jo. These were names people used to talk about right along with Jackie Robinson, who also had played for the Monarchs before he was signed by the Brooklyn Dodgers.

Watching the Monarchs was about the most fun you could have in Kansas City. Every Sunday what seemed like the entire black population of the city went directly from church services over to the ball park. The preachers tried to finish their preaching at one-thirty, in time so everyone could be in the park by two, which was when the national anthem was played. The place was jammed with people in high spirits, whites as well as blacks, many of them dressed up in their Sunday church clothes and ready for a party.

The money I made in Kansas City that summer helped me get

a start on the school year. But even with it the new semester started hard and proceeded to get harder. I had already switched to premed. But now I was determined to finish school as fast as I could. I figured out that if I took seven or eight subjects a semester and went to summer school too, I could graduate in three years instead of four. So I started out that year with a lot of courses: German again and English, and religion along with all the math and science I could squeeze in.

I also decided I didn't want to live in the dorms again. One way around that was that Philander Smith offered opportunities for students to live and work in people's homes. So that year, when I came back, I went out and started working for a black family in North Little Rock. I lived in, and they gave me room and board. In exchange I found myself taking care of not one house but two houses, this woman's and her daughter's house next door.

My employer sold products door to door, and her daughter and son-in-law owned a funeral home. I did the cleaning and cooking and dishes and washing and ironing, starch and all, which complicated things some and took time. It was a lot of work, and the two houses were a lot of work, and I also had all those courses to study for. On top of it, my employer wasn't the sympathetic sort. Her elderly crippled mother lived with her, and she was kinder. I think her mother felt I didn't have enough time for everything I had to do. Often when I'd get back from classes, she would have dinner already cooked, even though that was supposed to be my job. When her daughter would go on at me about something, she'd say, "Sister, sister, don't you talk to her like that."

But it didn't smooth things out much. Once my employer came home when I was studying for several big tests and asked me if I had finished some job. When I told her I was tired and had to study just then, she snapped, "Well, don't you think I get tired when I'm out there working to feed you?"

I stayed with her almost until the next summer, but it wasn't easy. As the year went on, other things began to pile up. The worst was that I was now pretty much out of touch with home.

I couldn't afford to go back for either Thanksgiving or Christmas, and while Mama and I wrote, her letters tended to be brief. "Dear Minnie," she'd say. "How are you? We're all fine. Daddy's fine. Katie is going to school every day and so is Charles." She'd write a sentence about each of them, then sign off.

In my heart I knew she and Daddy were thinking about me. But I wasn't feeling that they really understood. I was sure they didn't even know enough to know what kinds of problems I was having. Besides, they had all they could handle with the farm and with my younger sisters and brothers. Now that I was out, I couldn't expect they'd feel responsible for me too.

I didn't understand that I was going through a full-blown separation anxiety, which only got worse when Uncle Reva stopped sending money. Reva was one of my father's younger brothers. He was only five or six years older than I was, and I had known him my entire life. Reva had always been more like a troublemaking older brother than an uncle.

I say troublemaking, but what I really mean is mischievous— mischievous and funny and completely brazen. Uncle Reva was not your quiet, retiring type. Growing up, I played with him all the time. Even then he was always telling everybody what to do. Always getting into trouble and always getting other people in trouble. If some girl in school got her pigtails dunked in the inkwell, there was never a question about who had done it. Ree had. And loud? My whole family was always loud. We were constantly having to talk over a crowd. But he was even louder than the rest of us. He'd butt in and just take over a conversation. Everybody would say, "Oh, my God, here comes Reva. Nobody else'll get a word in." And whatever came up he knew more about it than everyone, even if he had never heard of it until that very moment it got mentioned.

In addition to his mischievousness and sense of fun, Reva had, and has, a heart of gold. It's not really surprising that he became a social worker later on in his life. He's married and has three grown children now. For years he used to talk about all the things he, for one, was not going to do for his kids. And at the very moment he was swearing he wasn't going to do a single one of them, he was doing them. With me he always took a protective attitude. If some boy was paying what he thought was too much attention, he'd say, "I'm not gonna let that ol' boy talk to you like that." And he wouldn't either.

By the time I got to college Ree was in the Army. But he kept in touch, and he used to send me money. He even tried to make out an allotment for my schooling, but the Army wouldn't let him do it. For some reason, during my second year Uncle Ree wasn't able to send anything for a while. Of course nothing was coming in from home either, which meant I didn't have a penny to my name. Plus there were some bills at the college that needed paying, and the only thing the secretaries who talked to me seemed to care about was collecting money I didn't have.

After struggling with this for a time, I got to feeling deserted. It began to seem to me that no one really cared about how I got by or even whether I could buy books or pencils. As far as I could see, nobody at all was worried or concerned in the least about what might happen to me.

One afternoon I was sitting on the long steps leading down from Philander Smith's administration building. I had just had another bad time with the secretaries. I can't remember if I was crying. But if I wasn't, I was close to it. I was just sitting there really downtrodden and sad. Obviously the people at the school didn't care if I stayed or went. Nobody else did either. Since I didn't have the money, I might as well just quit and go home. What was the use of trying to continue? I was already trying my hardest, but I was only getting deeper into this hole I was digging. It was beginning to look like maybe the time had just come to give it up.

While I was sniffling and wallowing around in that thought, Mr. Scott, the biology chairman, came walking up the steps. He had been my major professor in several courses, and we had gotten to know each other. Ever since I told him I was going to become a doctor, he had been trying to get me to take some education courses too, so I'd be able to get a teaching certificate. Just in case. Since I was sure I wasn't going to end up teaching, I kept refusing, but we had a kind of running discussion about it. Right at this moment, though, it was pretty clear to me how meaningless the argument was. I wasn't ever going to get to be either a doctor or a teacher.

When I told Mr. Scott what I had decided, he sat down beside me on the steps. He was a soft-spoken man, one of those people who never raise their voices and always speak at a level so you have to pay close attention and maybe cup your hand behind your ear to make sure you are catching it all. I was telling him that I was going to quit and I was going home, and he was saying in that low, steady voice, "Well, all right, so you've made up your mind. But tell me, exactly what are you going to do when you get back there? You planning to just work on the farm and chop and pick cotton and such?"

I said no, and he whispered, "Well then, what are you going to do?"

I told him I didn't know.

"I think we can find a way for you to stay here," he said. "I think we should try to get in there and work it out."

The details of how we eventually did work it out are lost. But I remember that Mr. Scott intervened with the bookkeepers to give me some breathing room and that eventually I was able to pay off the bills. What Mr. Scott really did was step in and give me encouragement when I was down and badly in need of it He got me over to the other side.

The next summer things got a little easier when I took a new live-in job with Mrs. Eva Morton, an older white lady who lived by herself in Edgehill, the wealthiest neighborhood in Little Rock. Philander Smith used to place a lot of girls in jobs at white homes. White families tended to like the idea of having a college student, and Methodists were happy to have someone from a Methodist college. Working for Mrs. Morton, I was taking care of only one house, and she was kind and understanding as far as my studies went. I stayed with her for the next year and a half, until I graduated. In fact she and her twin daughters, Mary and Martha, were my only guests at my graduation. Mama and Daddy would have loved to come, but when it came time, they couldn't afford the trip up.

Cornelius Reynolds was also at the graduation. Cornelius was a boy I had started seeing my junior year. He was a math major who had been a student assistant in a math course I was taking. Philander Smith was a strict place when it came to boys and girls. Boys were allowed into the girls' dormitory only on Friday and Saturday nights, and then they were restricted to the first-floor lounge area, next to where the dorm supervisor lived. They never, ever could go upstairs in the rooms. But there were football games and basketball games, and the college put on dances every once in a while. There was plenty of chance at Philander Smith for romance to develop.

Cornelius had started paying attention to me when I was a junior. One day he had seen me outside and had come over to ask how math was going. That started it. I had never really had anything like a boyfriend before. There had been a couple of boys in high school I liked, the kind you giggled about with your girlfriends but never actually got up the courage to say hello to. Besides, in Schaal there was no way to go out on anything that resembled a date, even if you did happen to start talking to someone. There had been one older boy who showed interest and had tried to come around. But my parents didn't like the idea, and Daddy made it clear he wasn't welcome. Since he wasn't about to challenge Daddy, he stopped.

Cornelius was really a nice young man, very courteous and kind, and we liked each other a lot. By the time I started getting near graduation we had been seeing each other for over a year and had decided to get married. Looking back, I wouldn't say this was a well-considered decision. Cornelius and I are still friends, and our brief time as a couple isn't one I think either he or I regard as a terrible period. But it's been many years since we've talked about it. Neither one of us was too happy in the relationship.

We got married in his hometown of Helena shortly after graduation. Helena is on the opposite side of Arkansas from Schaal, so my parents weren't able to come. I barely had time to see them before we moved up to Milwaukee, where Cornelius had gotten a job with the IRS. Life together wasn't awful, but from early on I think we both came to understand that the affection we had for each other wasn't strong enough to build a future on. At the same time I hadn't yet solved my main problem, which was how to get enough money to go to medical school. I had taken a job as a nurse's aide at the VA hospital. What I was able to save from my weekly earnings wasn't that much. But at least it was something, and I was keeping my eyes wide open for anything else that might come along.

One day I was walking along a street in downtown Milwaukee when I saw a sign advertising the Women's Medical Specialist Corps. If you were a college graduate, it said, you could join up to be trained as a physical therapist, speech therapist, or occupational therapist. The Army would send you to school and make you a commissioned officer.

That sounded interesting. When I went into the recruiting office, they told me about the training I'd get if I joined up. Once I was certified as a therapist, the Army would also pay for college courses if I wanted to take any. Plus, when I finished school, I'd be a second lieutenant with a second lieutenant's salary, a lot more than I was making as a nurse's aide. Then came the capper: I'd also be eligible for the GI Bill. For every year I spent in the service the government would give me a year's worth of financial credits toward my education.

I couldn't believe what I had stumbled on. It sounded too good to be true. If I stayed in three years, that would be good for thirty-six months' worth of medical school. My mind was calculating a mile a minute. Thirty-six months was about four years' worth of school. If I did this, it looked like the Army would pay my whole tuition. And once I got into medical school, I'd work summers, of course, so I could make money to live on. This thing looked like it could be the answer.

I signed up then and there. I didn't even tell Cornelius about it until right before I was about to leave for training. I didn't want to be married, and neither did he, so working things out with him didn't seem like a priority. I think we both understood that my going into the Army would finish the marriage. He would be in Milwaukee, and I would be wherever the Army wanted me to be. We didn't talk about divorce, and it was awhile before we actually got one, but that was really the end of our being married right there.

The morning after I told Cornelius I got on a train for Brooke Army Medical Center in San Antonio, Texas. This was in May 1953. The U.S. Army had been desegregated since Truman's order in 1948. I knew that. But I didn't know how extremely few black women there were in the new desegregated Army. When I arrived at the huge Fort Sam Houston, where the Brooke Army Center was, I seemed to be the only one. When I met my training class, I found it was seventeen young white women and me.

Chapter 6

More Than Most

Brooke Army Center might not have been paradise on earth, but it was as close to it as I had ever come. My seventeen classmates were from all over: Illinois, Alabama, California, Tennessee, north, south, east, and west. This was the first time I had been in school with whites since California. I can't say I was apprehensive, but I did wonder what it was going to be like. Right from the first, though, they struck me as really bright and well educated and friendly. The way the school worked we did everything as a group, and we all just seemed to hit it off from the start. The classes weren't much different from college, except that they went from eight to five every day. Mornings we had lectures; then in the afternoon we practiced what we were learning, using each other as subjects. We ate together, and after dinner we studied together to get ready for the next day.

We had classes in anatomy, physiology, kinesiology, exercise physiology, and other subjects, so the work load was heavy. But compared with what I was used to, physical therapy school was more enjoyment than anything else. At Philander Smith just plain surviving had been such a struggle. Now the only thing anybody wanted me to do was sit and study. No more scrubbing or washing or ironing. No more worrying all the time how I was going to scrape up money to pay my bills. Instead of that,

I was the one who was getting paid. I felt like I had joined the middle class.

To make things even better, from early on I knew I was going to love physical therapy. I liked working with people. And after a while I realized that I had a feel for physical problems and that I was good with my hands. It felt good helping patients learn to do the necessities for themselves, whether it was walking or eating or bathing or something else.

After six months' training I was sent off for an internship at Letterman Army Hospital in San Francisco. This was in October 1953. Letterman had the usual peacetime injuries, but the Korean War had ended only in July, and the hospital was still full of battle casualties. Young men who had lost hands or arms or legs were there. Many had spinal injuries and were paralyzed from the waist or the neck down.

It wasn't easy seeing so many boys more or less my own age who were badly hurt. But by the time they started physical therapy most of them had begun adjusting to their injuries. Almost always they were hard at work trying to regain whatever abilities they could. What you mainly got from them was a feeling of determination and hope. They were in bad shape, but they were alive. And they knew that they could help themselves if only they stuck to it.

I'd have someone come to me sitting in a wheelchair, who couldn't even get out of it alone, couldn't stand up, couldn't walk at all, couldn't go to the bathroom by himself. With enough work I could get him up and have him standing and walking and using crutches and going to the bathroom and getting in the bathtub without help. That was something to watch. I thought that the feeling it gave me was probably a lot like the feeling you'd get from doctoring.

At the end of my six-month internship at Letterman I took the exam and became a licensed physical therapist, which meant I was certified to practice on my own. As soon as I had my license, the Army transferred me to Fitzsimmons Hospital in Denver, a huge facility of probably two thousand beds. Fitzsimmons was a general hospital, but it took many acute cases and did lots and lots of rehabilitation.

At Fitzsimmons the percentage of war wounded wasn't as high as at Letterman, but otherwise the work was more or less the same. My routine did break, though, when I and another therapist were sent one day to take care of President Dwight Eisenhower. After his heart attack they had brought Ike to Fitzsimmons, which of course was the talk of the place. Given how big the hospital was, I never expected to see him, let alone treat him. But there I was, standing in his room one morning, saying, "Mr. President, we're here to do the exercises that your doctor ordered."

"Well, go ahead then," he said. That was pretty nearly all he did say while we manipulated his arms and legs, giving him what are called range-of-motion exercises.

The word on Eisenhower was that he was a charming gentleman. I think he was, but it was a little hard to judge. The days we were in there with him it was obvious he was not really feeling that well. He did what we told him, and when we were through exercising him, he thanked us. But it was more an "I'm so glad you're through" kind of thanks.

Being a medical specialist in the Army wasn't a bad life. There was no real regimentation. Other than the requirements of the job I was free to come and go as I pleased. I loved the work, and I liked Colorado a lot. The Rockies had looked so beautiful to me when I crossed them at the age of twelve on that train, and they still did. I made some hiking and camping excursions, and I promised myself I'd learn to ski, though I never quite got around to that. A lot of my colleagues were planning careers in the service. Under different circumstances I could have stayed in the Army as a physical therapist forever. Actually that thought would have had some real attractiveness if I hadn't been so completely set on going to medical school. If anything, as my third year in the Army got under way and I could see my GI Bill benefits accumulating, I got more excited about it than ever.

During that year I took the M-CATs and applied to schools. I was accepted at the University of Colorado, Meharry Medical College, and the University of Arkansas. I liked living in Colorado, and Meharry was the premier black medical school, so that was an incentive, but Arkansas was home. It was also the cheapest by far, $270 a semester. So when it came down to it, the decision wasn't hard. When my enlistment came up in May, I resigned my commission and got a temporary position at the VA hospital in Oklahoma City. In September I was back in Little Rock.

The entering class of 1956 at the University of Arkansas Medical School had about one hundred students. Three were black, and three were women. I was the only one who was both. There had been a number of other black medical students at Arkansas since Edith Irby, including Henry Foster, who was a third-year student when I entered. But I was only the second black female.

Of course the three black students quickly got to know one another well. Bobby Mims, William Mays, and I tended to study together and we had a kind of natural solidarity. But we didn't feel isolated from our classmates or treated differently by our professors. I didn't, and I'm pretty sure they didn't either. We had friends, and we interacted with everybody. I understand that other black students, even long after my time, may have had different experiences, but if there was any sniping going on against me, I wasn't aware of it.

The only institutional discrimination left at the med school when I got there was the cafeteria, which was whites only. Black medical students could not eat in the white lunchroom, which meant that we took our meals with the black hospital staff in their cafeteria. The three of us and the cleaning people and nurse's aides and maybe a few nurses, though I'm not sure I remember many black nurses from that period. I know there were no black doctors.

Had there been, the lunchroom situation might have turned interesting. As it was, the three of us were right at home with the hospital's black workers. Also, we all understood that the aim of this game was to get through medical school. Right from the start we were far more concerned with that than we were with something like where we ate. By the time I got ready to go to lunch I didn't have a lot of interest in trying to integrate the dining room. What I wanted after a hard morning of classes was to sit down with some of my friends and relax, which I could do at least as well in the black cafeteria.

Besides, this was old news. I was born and raised in the South, where we never really had been a part of that other society. All of us had gone around to the back door to eat. Or to the colored restaurants, if you ever actually went to a restaurant. In fact the best black restaurant in Little Rock was also one of the best white restaurants. Whit's Cafe had a black side and a white side, both served by the same kitchen. I had never gone there in college, but I did when I came back to medical school, and when I ate there, I wasn't thinking about the white folks eating on the other side of the wall. I was thinking about how great it was to have money to do something like this in the first place.

Looking back on all this now, I wonder if I didn't just block out the antagonism that came with a segregated society because I had developed such a tough crust when I was younger. Oliver thinks that's so, and he might see it more clearly than I. He will talk about what happens to you on a farm when you're the oldest and you have the responsibility to get this amount chopped or that amount picked regardless of the hundred other things that might be bothering you. He's done his own share of farm work, so he knows what it's like to be out in the mosquitoes and the heat. It makes a person hard—that's his opinion. It trains you to slough off the unessentials and put your whole mind into what needs to get done. I know this isn't the entire story, but there's probably more than a grain of truth to it.

There are certainly things I remember with a kind of strange equanimity, the lunchroom being one. Another was an incident that happened with my roommate Lillyann Farley and me. Lillyann was a white girl whom I knew slightly from Colorado, where we had taken our M-CATs together. We were living in a duplex that was right on the dividing line between black and white Little Rock. Actually we lived on the black side of the line, but our backyard abutted on the white side. At one point a group of white neighbors came by to let Lillyann know that they didn't consider it right or proper for her to be living with a black person. They wanted her to do something about it.

Fine, said Lillyann, but she had signed a lease. Were they saying they were offering to pay for her to live somewhere else? That was the end of anyone asking her to move, as Lillyann knew it would be. I watched all this without any real anger or upset. More than anything I was curious as to how Lillyann was going to handle it. How these people could have had the effrontery for such a thing didn't particularly interest me.

It was the rare incident that got through my crust. But it's true that some did. One of those happened later that year at the med school. A group of us were talking with some doctors about an experiment that had not turned out the way it was supposed to. No one was sure what had gone wrong, but it was clear that something must have. "Well," one of the doctors said, shaking his head, "you just know there's got to be a nigger in the woodpile somewhere."

I looked up and stared directly at him. I didn't say a word, just stared. The room was dead silent. And somehow right in the middle of it I felt that I needed to save this person. "Well," I said, "I guess we have to keep digging till we find the results." Then somebody else said something, and we moved away from it. It was like a rescue operation.

The next day the professor who had made the remark came to apologize. It was just an expression, he said, something he used without thinking. He was sorry; he hadn't meant to offend me. I thought, well, I hadn't liked hearing it, but I wasn't exactly mortally wounded either. This was the kind of thing that could make you uncomfortable for a moment, but it wasn't Bull Connor. Neither was it Silas Hunt listening to lectures from behind some boards.

There was maybe one other incident like that I recall in my four years of medical school in Arkansas. And that wasn't meant viciously either. One of my professors, a woman OB-GYN, was telling me how much she liked my work. She meant to give me a compliment, but what came out was "You know, you have as much education as a lot of white people." I don't know what in the world could have been going through her head; I was already a fourth-year medical student at that point. I remember I said to her, "Doctor, I have more education than *most* white people."

I remember this now, just like I do the "nigger in the wood-pile" business. So there's no doubt they made an impression. But I'm not sure I saw them as any big thing. I didn't nurse them. We probably had lots of incidents like this happening that I don't even remember. The thing was, if you let yourself get bogged down in resentment, you would never get anything done at all. You'd be paralyzed.

That was true even during my second year, 1957. That was the year Little Rock's Central High School was integrated. My apartment wasn't far from there, and two of the kids who had been chosen for it lived just a couple of blocks from me. Mrs. Daisy Bates, the woman who had given Edith Irby the money she needed to make up her tuition, lived nearby too. It was Daisy and her husband, L.C., who were the driving force behind the integration fight.

I knew her, like everyone in the black community did. She was probably forty then, a warm, loving woman who also knew how to stand up and be counted. Daisy Bates drew controversy; she encouraged it. She would just say what she felt needed to be said, no matter how controversial it might have seemed to somebody else. You would hear her, and even though you agreed with her 100 percent, you'd find yourself thinking, Why did she have to come out and say that? But she was out there with the children facing those mobs, and she was giving speeches all around the country. Her husband ran the newspaper and wrote articles, and she took care of the activist side.

So I knew her, but I didn't take part in the struggle. What I saw of it—the crowds attacking the nine black children, Orval Faubus's National Guard protecting the white rioters, the federal troops when they arrived—I saw on television. But I didn't even see that much, and I can't say that I appreciated the importance of it all. What I understood better was that I was drowning in work, which was true not just of me but of all the first- and second-year students. If I was going to get through what I personally had in front of me, I didn't have a lot of time or energy to spend on other things. It wasn't a question of choosing. Even without distractions I had more to do than I had time to do it in. So while Daisy Bates and Martin Luther King and Thurgood Marshall were out fighting all over the South, I was keeping my nose in my books studying medicine.

The year I started, the medical school had just finished its new buildings and was in the process of moving. Because of that, the usual routine of studies was a little different for my class. Ordinarily there'd be science lectures in the morning and biochemistry and anatomy labs in the afternoon. But the new anatomy labs weren't ready yet, so the administration decided to get all our anatomy work in while the old labs were still available. That meant jamming a year's worth of anatomy into a semester.

That was why for four hours a day four days a week I was hunched over a cadaver with three of my white classmates, dissecting out parts. This was a situation that made you learn to like one another, a lot. You were responsible for showing the others in your group what you were doing, and they were responsible for showing you. So if you couldn't get along and work together, you all were in deep trouble. In anatomy lab it was strictly all for one and one for all.

Once I got over the smell of formaldehyde, working on the cadaver wasn't at all troubling. What inevitably happens is that you begin to develop a kind of relationship; you aren't in any way negative. After a while it becomes your own cadaver, and you feel very friendly toward him, even protective and a little emotional.

Ours was a white male, though white or black didn't mean any more to us than it did to him at that point. Once you get through the skin, the very first thing you do in anatomy lab, it's all the same. You cut through the skin. Then you make your way through every individual layer, from head to toe and top to bottom. You take out each muscle, each blood vessel; you identify it, label it, and learn its name. Ordinarily it takes two semesters to do this. We did it in one. We learned the structures; we traced them from origin to terminus; we learned what was above, below, and on either side of them. We dissected them out. We got to where we could go to any structure in the body at any time, on our own, without looking at the labels that identified parts in our laboratory's comparison cadaver.

Many medical students feel a little sick when they see their first operations or patients with certain gross manifestations. I didn't, maybe in part because of my experience as a physical therapist. I had already seen and dealt with a lot of upsetting difficulties. The one time I did have to go and sit down was when we were treating a woman who had just delivered a baby and was hemorrhaging profusely. A river of blood was flowing out, and the doctors were working furiously to stop it. I could feel myself getting nauseated and shaky, and finally I just had to walk away. But that experience never repeated itself, fortunately, because like everyone else, I started finding myself regularly around blood and deaths of every description.

Physical therapy may have given me an advantage in learning anatomy, at least the muscles, bones, and joints, but it didn't help at all with biochemistry or physiology or microbiology. Medical school was a challenge, no question, and stressful. You got completely immersed in it. It absolutely required that of you.

So that's where I was while Central High was being fought: immersed and stressed out. But though I might not have been too conscious of it, what was happening in Montgomery and Little Rock and elsewhere in the South didn't just leave me untouched. I realized that when I went home to Schaal for a visit and found myself doing something that surprised me and horrified my brothers and sisters.

While I was in the Army, I had bought a television set for Mama and Daddy. I could do that because rural electrification had reached the farms in Howard County, probably when I was in college. The family had gotten a radio then, which put them in touch with the world outside Schaal in a way we never were when I was growing up. Once I had some money coming in, I kept an eye out for what appliances I could buy them, and at some point I had acquired this television set.

I didn't know it, but in 1957 the Walt Disney company was advertising like crazy on children's television shows for its big new movie *Old Yeller*. The result of that was that my brothers and sisters, the ones who were still at home, wanted to see this movie more than they wanted presents for Christmas. The first I ever heard of *Old Yeller* was when I drove home in my new lavender and white Pontiac to visit. But once I got there I never heard the end of it. With everyone jabbering away about it non-stop, I finally decided to pile them all into the car and take them up to the Nashville drive-in where it was playing.

Had I been a little more tuned in, I would have understood what all the fuss was, other than the fact that this was a popular hit movie. But I wasn't. I didn't even have any idea exactly what *Old Yeller* was about, other than some dog. For my little brothers and sisters, though, the advertisements had made this dog out to be an exact reincarnation of Old Don, our wonderful bulldog, who had died not very long before.

For people who don't remember or maybe never saw *Old Yeller,* it's about a big dog that attaches itself to the children of a pioneer farming family in Texas. While their father is away, Old Yeller takes care of the children. He saves them from snakes and fights wolves and hunts the family's wild pigs, which slash him so badly he almost dies. There's even a scene where the little farm boy rides around on his back. All this was like a duplicate picture of Old Don. I don't know if they shot that movie in Texas or where, but even the countryside looked like ours. In the end Old Yeller gets rabies from a mad wolf he has fought off and the older farm boy has to take his father's shotgun and shoot him, his best friend in the world. Even for ordinary people this movie is a tearjerker. For our crew the advertising previews had put them in a state.

I didn't know any of this. All I knew was I was taking them out to the drive-in. But Chester knew. He was thirteen then, and the thought of seeing this movie had him spinning out of control. "I tell you"—this is Chester now, talking about *Old Yeller*—"if you want to understand something about what happened in our lives, you need to see that movie. That was our own theme. It was absolutely crucial for us to see it. After Old Don died, that was our therapy."

Anyway, I took the carful of them up to Nashville without understanding what I had gotten into the middle of. When we got to the drive-in, there weren't many other people there. The white section up front was nearly empty, and so was the colored section in back. I don't know exactly what happened to me when I saw that. Maybe it was that I had been living as a free and independent adult for three or four years now, or maybe being a medical student had given me a feeling that I was probably as good as anybody else. Then again, by that time Rosa Parks had entered like an icon into everybody's mind, mine included. Whatever it was, when I saw all those empty spaces up front near the screen, I just drove up and parked the car there.

When they realized what I was doing, my brothers and sisters went totally silent, which was a big contrast with the kind of noise they had been filling the car with the whole ride up. I guess I was aware of that, but I wasn't particularly thinking about them at that point. I was thinking that I had paid my money and I was damned if I was going to park back there in the Negro section when there were all these places up close. Nobody had even said anything to me yet, but I was already steaming. Had I bothered to look at my brothers and sisters, I would have seen cold terror in their eyes. Chester said later that he thought being up in the city for so long had caused me to lose my mind.

Then the attendant came over to tell me we weren't allowed to sit up there. That was all I needed to hear. I was so upset I didn't know what to do. It was for sure I was not going to park back there in the back. When I got unflustered enough to say something, I told him, fine, I wanted my money back because I was leaving. When they heard this, everyone in the car broke out crying. It was like opening a spigot. They wanted to see *Old Yeller* so bad they would have watched it from across the street with a spyglass.

Finally I just couldn't bear them taking on like that. So I drove the car around to the area between the black and white sections and sort of perched it on the edge. Like a dare. I don't know what I would have done had the attendant come to tell me to move back farther, but he didn't. I was so angry I refused to watch the movie. Of course Chester and the others were enthralled. They were seeing their lives unfold up there on the screen. It was my life up there as well as theirs, but I had made enough concessions for one day.

—

As opposed to the first two years, my third year in medical school was a pleasure. That was when you got to go out on the wards and see patients. That meant you could start to feel that you were a doctor, someone important, even if you really weren't quite. After sitting in classrooms for two years, I was ready.

Third-year students worked in teams. We were assigned patients whom we saw during the day, and we'd be on night call as well. I'd ordinarily get to the hospital at six in the morning, work till nine at night, then be on call after that. In those days they had senior med students doing things they wouldn't think of having them do today. We spent a lot of time running around doing blood work-ups and urine analyses and EKGs, things technicians do far better than apprentice doctors. But we were the ones who did them then, as well as everything else the residents told us to do. We were like super ward aides.

At Arkansas, like most medical schools, third- and fourth-year students go on rotations, spending time on each of the hospital's services: medicine, surgery, pediatrics, OB-GYN, neurology, psychiatry, and the others. My problem was that every service I went on, that's what I wanted to be. I can't recall a rotation I didn't like. So even when I became a senior, I was still wondering what I wanted to be when I grew up, at least in terms of choosing a specialty.

One of the real power brokers at Arkansas University Hospital was Dr. James Growdon, chief of surgery. Along with two or three other chiefs of services, he dominated the medical school landscape. Everyone thought of him as the world's worst grouch—when they were feeling charitable. He had that kind of typical surgeon's attitude, short on temper and long on abuse. He was a tall, imposing man and a tyrant. If he wasn't screaming at residents and nurses and throwing things around, they would have thought they were in the wrong operating room.

But he was a masterful surgeon. He was famous for his meticulousness and control of blood loss. It was said that all the Seventh-Day Adventists who needed operations came to him since their beliefs didn't allow for blood transfusions.

It was hard to say for sure, but I had the impression that he was taking a special interest in me. He always made sure that during his operations I was positioned right to see everything, and he seemed pleased with my work and the fact that I took pains to know my patients. For my part, I was mesmerized. When he started operating, his concentration set him off from everyone around him. He always seemed so careful, so very intense and precise that it was as if he had slipped into another world. The surgical lights were glaring down, the rows of instruments were gleaming on the trays, and he'd be towering there in the middle with all his surgeon's paraphernalia on. Out of whatever zone he was in he'd call for instruments, and the nurses knew exactly what he needed. They'd slap them into his hand even while he was naming them, like choreography. When Dr. Growdon operated, there was a mystique in the room you could feel.

The entire time he'd be talking about what he was doing. "Now we're going to cut here through the skin. Now we're moving through this tissue. We're getting down to the first layer; you can see it there. We're going to go down, down deep. Near nerve territory now, watch it. Come with me now; don't cover up your field." He wasn't really talking to you, yet he was talking directly to you, teaching you and showing you, sometimes for six or eight or ten hours at a stretch, however long the operation took. And through the whole thing he never lost his concentration, whether he was sailing right along or erupting into some roaring tantrum when someone did something she or he shouldn't have.

After the first couple of days on surgical rounds, Growdon and the other surgeons let the students assist. We did prep work on the patients and held clamps. Eventually they let us open up the skin or sew incisions closed when an operation was finished. I was getting used to doing these minor bits of surgery when one day during an appendectomy Growdon said, "Okay, Joycelyn, I want you to isolate that appendix up there so we can take it out."

I was startled, not only because this was an unusual thing for a student to do, but because I was halfway in a reverie when he said it. The patient was a five- or six-year-old boy with a ruptured appendix. I had seen him up on the pediatric ward when they first brought him in, sick as a dog, with his stomach swollen and hard. The instant I saw him I thought of Bernard, that this was exactly what he had had. I remembered my father's voice when he brought Bernard back on the mule that night and told us, "The doctor said his appendix burst."

Now we had this little boy opened up on the table, and I was staring at a hot, necrotic appendix, already turning black and dying. The moment when Growdon said, "I want you to isolate it," I was having flashbacks of Bernard. I was thinking, So this is what was wrong, this is what it looks like. Then he said a little more urgently, "You have to get it all the way out so we can really see it."

Nestled up there against the pink peritoneum, the bowel was grayish and loaded with blood vessels, like the bowel of a chicken, I thought. Or chitlins in a hog. Large and wormy, even in this little boy, with reddish blood vessels and lots of ivory-colored fat. I was now supposed to lift this section of the bowel up onto the surgical draping so we could snip it off its poisonous little black appendage without spilling any more matter into the interior.

I could see the viscous yellow pus floating on the inflamed peritoneum. This boy was infected, but he wasn't in septic shock yet. Bernard couldn't have been either, I thought. In septic shock there is a marked dilation of the vessels out into the extremities and a pooling of blood. There was none of that yet. Everything was prepared. All the connecting structures were sectioned, sutured, and clamped. I got my hands under the bowel and lifted, then laid it carefully onto the sterile cloth.

Well! There were other formidable characters among my professors. But at that moment there wasn't one of them ahead of Dr. Growdon in my personal pantheon. As the semester went on, I began to think I might even have the hands for surgery. I liked delicate work. In some ways it reminded me of embroidery. I was good at "cut downs," making tiny incisions in children's veins and threading in IV catheters, then suturing above and below to hold it steady. Before long they were asking me to do all of those.

I was inclined toward surgery, not just the physical side of it but the emotional. Surgeons are quick-fix people. They like the idea of curing problems now. They want to identify the cause and attack it head-on, as opposed, for example, to psychiatrists, who tend to think in long terms and incremental improvements. No question I had a lot more of the surgeon in me than the psychiatrist. But Dr. Growdon wasn't the only professor who attracted me. Another powerhouse at the medical school was Ted Panos, chief of pediatrics. And Dr. Panos was recruiting me hard to take a pediatric internship.

Panos was an extraordinary teacher with a powerful, wide-ranging intellect. You didn't find too many doctors who were also intellectuals. But knowledge for him went way beyond the confines of medicine. Before deciding on medical school, he had studied theology and languages, which he was still up on and liked to discuss. He knew Spanish and Latin and ancient Greek, and he was studying Russian. He loved art too, and the classics, which he read in the original. The pediatrics library looked like it had as many classics in it as medical books. One of the staff doctors told us that if we ever got bored doing medicine, we could go in there and read up on Greek mythology.

Later I got to know Panos well. His dad was a Greek immigrant who had worked building the Union Pacific Railroad until he made enough money and stopped. By that time he was out in Wyoming, so that's where he stayed.

Though Panos himself wasn't born in Greece, he grew up speaking Greek, and I always thought he had some sort of little accent, which he hid by speaking in a clipped kind of way. He took great pride in his diction. He chose his words with care. He liked me, and because he did, he thought nothing of calling me into his office to point out that I was saying "was" when I should be using "were," or maybe "good" when "well" was more proper. He was extremely delicate about this. He did it in a way that didn't make me feel bad. But he definitely wanted me to know. I wasn't offended. I took it for what it was, an expression of friendship and protectiveness. He wanted me to succeed and he thought the way would be easier if my grammar were better.

Dr. Panos wanted me to stay at Arkansas. But there was a young staff pediatrician named Rosalind Abernathy who began talking to me about doing a pediatric internship at the University of Minnesota. Everybody knew that the two best pediatric slots in the country were at Boston Children's Hospital and Minnesota. Rosalind had done her own residency at Minnesota and so had her husband, Robert, an internist who some years later became chairman of medicine at Arkansas.

According to Rosalind, the Minnesota pediatric department had some idiosyncrasies in the way they chose interns. They never took two interns from the same school, she said, regardless of how good they were. Since the department more or less had the pick of the medical school crop, they put an emphasis on geographical and other kinds of diversity. They would for sure be looking to take someone from the South. And here I was, a black female southerner. If I applied, I'd give them a chance to kill three birds with one stone. What's more, supposedly Minnesota gave special weight to recommendations from their former

students, and both Rosalind and her husband would be pushing me.

I liked surgery, but I was drawn to pediatrics too. At the time
I never bothered to analyze my attraction, except maybe that
young patients added a notch of difficulty to diagnostic problems, so there was that extra challenge. But looking at it now,
I can see there might have been more to it. After all, what had
I done my entire young life from the age of four on but take
care of children? It wasn't just Bernard's appendicitis that left
an impression. It was watching over dozens of other only slightly
less severe injuries and sicknesses my sisters and brothers suffered through, all of them with no help from medicine. None
of that occurred to me at the time, not overtly anyway. But I
wonder now if it might not have been underneath in some form
all along.

What pushed me over the line was Dr. Panos. He had also
studied at Minnesota, and he thought it would be all right if I
did an internship there. Then I could come back to Arkansas
for my residency. So he'd support my application there too. I
also understood that studying pediatrics didn't necessarily mean
giving up surgery. Pediatric surgery was a relatively new specialty. It was something I could shoot for.

———

The University of Minnesota was interested and scheduled interviews for me over the Christmas break. This was an exciting
development. The uncertainty I had been feeling about the future started going away. Minnesota had a good ring to it. A bit
cold, maybe, but I had spent two years in the Rockies, so a little
snow wasn't going to kill me. The main thing was that if the
university took me, I'd be set. My life seemed to be laying itself
out in just the nice orderly way I wanted it to.

In the meantime I went about my business, part of which was
a visit over to Horace Mann, Little Rock's only black high
school. One of the services the medical school provided was giving physical examinations to high school sports teams whose ath-
letes needed them before they were allowed to compete.

Ordinarily fourth-year students were sent out to do these, and my turn had come up. I was going over to Horace Mann to look at the basketball team. I was supposed to find the coach first, someone named Oliver Elders. He was the one who would get me set up with the players.

Chapter 7

Talking Death

When I walked in the door of Horace Mann and looked into the gym, it was a madhouse. Balls were bouncing and echoing, and lots of boys were running around playing basketball. I hadn't really thought about it until that moment, but when I looked in and saw them, it struck me that a bunch of adolescent boys might be nervous about being checked over by a woman doctor. I didn't think there would be a problem, but the thought did pass through my mind. Oliver of course saw the situation from the other side, close up. This is how he remembers what happened.

Oliver: "Each year the coaches would call the medical center. They'd send doctors out, and we'd give them a season pass for the basketball or football games or whatever was going on. So when we called that year, they said they'd have a doctor out there, and we should just keep an eye out.

"We hadn't had practice yet that day, and I was wanting to get it on. We had an important game coming up. So I told one of the boys to stay by the door and usher the doctor in. To make it faster, I was going to have all the guys strip down, and all they'd have to do is just line up and step through and be quick, so we could get started.

"A little later, when I looked over to the door, I saw this lady in navy blue with a bag talking with my player. He was probably telling her that the office was upstairs, but she just sort of stood there. I hadn't noticed this lady before. I had never seen her around. But all these guys were about half naked, and she was just standing there looking in.

"So I walked over and said, 'Ma'am, the office is a couple doors up and you just turn to the left. Somebody up there can help you.' And she said, 'You asked for a doctor, didn't you? If you want these guys examined, I'm the doctor.' Well, my mouth was open, and I couldn't close it, because up till then I had literally never heard of a lady doctor. I thought that doctors were males per se. We had always had men. And so I just thought, Oh Lord, what in the world? But after a bit I said, 'All right, let me go over there and get these guys.'

"So I blew my whistle. I was hot. I brought all the guys up, and I told them, 'All right, heads up. Listen up. The doctor's here to give her exam, and that's her right there.' And man, there was pandemonium. They all started going, 'Not me. No, sir. She's not going to be touching me!' It took me awhile to get them calmed down, and the way I finally did was that I said, 'Well, I'm going to be the first one to go through.'

"Of course I didn't have to take the exam myself, but the coaches often did. I always got a physical whenever the doctor came down; that was my yearly checkup. So I went through, and then the guys finally lined up, and they went through. Well, Joycelyn was just a big hit with them. She had this way of being friendly and reassuring. She'd engage them. She'd say, 'You're a strong young man. You look like you're going to be a good basketball player for Coach Elders. How do you feel?' And they were going, 'Yes, ma'am. Yes, ma'am.' She just kind of embraced them and got a dialogue going with them."

———

Once they started coming into the office I was using as an examination room, there were no problems. The funny thing is, I remember the kids pushing and jostling one another, probably trying to avoid being next, and I remember Oliver telling them,

"Go on in there. It's your turn. You're next." But I don't have any recollection of examining Oliver himself, which you'd think might be the one thing I would remember.

Oliver says that afterward he gave me my pass and invited me to come and see the basketball games. He says that he never actually expected that I would come but that at the first game he saw me in the stands, looking down at him. He says that he nodded at me, to acknowledge that I was there, and that I nodded back. But at the end of the game when he looked for me, I had gone. He says the same thing happened one or two more times, that he would see me in the stands, then I'd disappear. That's his version.

Now, it's a fact that I was interested. I'm not saying I wasn't. I had noticed Oliver the first moment I walked into that gym. As tall and handsome as he was, it would have been hard not to. But that isn't the way I remember it. The way I remember it is that Oliver did not give me the pass. Instead, when I was finished examining his boys, we got to talking, and he told me about the first game that was coming up. When I said I thought I might like to come, he said, "Well, I've got a pass for you. Could I come and pick you up?" That's the true story of how I started my career as a basketball fan.

I took up my interest in basketball sometime in November, and in mid-December I had to go up to Minneapolis for my interviews. When I told Oliver, he said, "Well, would you like me to drive you?" Now just a day or two before this he had told me that he was going to go over to Memphis to take the girl he was going out with to a dance.

So I said, "Oh, that would really be nice. But how are you going to explain to your girlfriend that you've got time to drive me to Minneapolis but you don't have time to drive her to Memphis?"

And he told me, "Don't worry. I'll take care of that." So I knew then that I didn't have to worry too much about this girlfriend.

Oliver did drive me up to Minnesota, and by the time we got back we were making plans to stay together. Two months later, on Valentine's Day 1960, we were married by Reverend Morley of the Liberty Hills Baptist Church, where Oliver's landlady, Mrs. Harris, was a member.

After that I moved into the room Oliver was renting at the Harrises' house not far from Horace Mann High School. We both had extra full schedules. Oliver was teaching and coaching, which kept him late most nights, and I was in my last semester at the medical school, which is like a definition of never having a free moment. As busy as we were, living at the Harrises was perfect. Mrs. Harris was a wonderful cook and prepared all the meals, in addition to doing the cleaning and laundry. Technically I guess we were roomers, but she treated Oliver and me as if we were her children. It was like going home and living with your mother.

Even though we were just married, we already had a separation coming up. The University of Minnesota had told me after my interviews that if I would rank them first on my list of preferences, they would accept me as a pediatric intern. The result was that I got the appointment and would have to leave for Minneapolis in June, as soon as I graduated. We both hated the idea of separating, especially Oliver, whose parents' jobs had kept them apart for a time when he was young. But we both knew that an internship there would be the best thing in the long run for the family we were going to have. Oliver was ready to make any sacrifice at all for that cause. I was too. But I also thought that if I had known I was going to fall in love with someone whose career was in Arkansas, I most likely never would have even thought about Minnesota.

When I started with Oliver, basketball was not something I knew a lot about. But I remedied that fast. Spending time with Oliver, you became a student of the sport. From the beginning of that season to the end I don't think I missed a game. I'm not sure how I did that, given what I was involved in at the medical school. But somehow I managed. I traded on-call nights with people, even if sometimes I had to give up two nights for one game night. I worked crazy hours. And I went. Sometimes Oliver would even come by the hospital to pick me up in the team bus. Or we'd meet out on the highway somewhere. I'd leave the car over by the side of the road and get on that bus. But I'd be there. I got involved.

Oliver hadn't been coaching too long at Horace Mann, but he had been a famous player and was already well on his way to becoming a famous coach. In Arkansas that was saying something. Football is big here, but basketball came before football to most of the state, and in many places it was *the* great attraction. If you've seen the movie *Hoosiers,* about high school basketball in small-town Indiana, you know what it was like in Arkansas, except doubled. Years later, when I was appointed director of public health, Oliver was already the winningest high school coach in Arkansas history. The way the media introduced me to the public was by identifying me as Coach Elders's wife. To this day Oliver is more widely recognized in Arkansas than I am. And except for me there probably isn't anyone in the entire state who calls him Oliver. Everyone calls him Coach.

Oliver was from De Witt, a rice-growing town in the delta. Both his parents were teachers—his mother in elementary and his father in high school, first as a teacher, then as principal. By the time they retired they had a hundred years of teaching experience between them. They were the kind of people who were pillars of their community, just as our teachers back in Howard County were. They did people's income taxes, kept their books, helped them file for Social Security or fill out their papers if they had been drafted.

Oliver's father was Oliver senior, but he was universally called Prof. I never once saw him without a tie and jacket until after he and Oliver's mother, Leona, moved in with us thirty years later in their advanced old age. Oliver claims that some friend once persuaded his father to wear a sport shirt instead of his suit, and everyone in De Witt, white and black, was doing a double take.

Oliver himself grew up a brilliant athlete. He was a diver and a gymnast and a swimmer and the quarterback on his high school football team. But basketball was his game. Twice his high school was state champs while he was captain, and once they went to the national championships. Then he got a scholarship to AM&N, which later became the University of Arkansas at Pine Bluff. Since his two older sisters had gone to AM&N before him, he was known there as Little Elders.

Oliver was the point guard. People who saw him play say he was quick as spit and could shoot your eyes out. AM&N won one conference championship while he was there and was runner-up for another. They were the biggest thing in ten counties. That whole part of the state used to flock to their games. Of course, I didn't know any of this when I first met him, and Oliver doesn't do any bragging at all. But over the years I got to know the story, partly from him and partly from people like Joyce Montgomery, my dear friend and college roommate who is his cousin and grew up in the same area. Later he played professionally with the Harlem Magicians until he ruptured an Achilles tendon, which ended his playing days.

Oliver started coaching and teaching after being in the Army a couple of years. He coached first at Emmanuel High School in Almyra, which was a backcountry area populated by his cousins, including the Montgomerys. A lot of them were tall and could play, so most of Oliver's team down there were his younger relatives. They were called the Zebras and wore black-and-white-striped uniforms. When they went up to Little Rock for the big tournament, they were so country that people laughed at them out loud.

What folks in Little Rock didn't know was that Oliver's Zebras were ballplayers and that Oliver was a different kind of coach. Oliver brought fast-break basketball to Arkansas. At that time all the others were still walking the ball up the court and passing fifteen or twenty times before they shot, which was the old style of playing. But Oliver's team ran up the court. He surprised them. Then on defense they pressed the whole game. Oliver used to say his boys would pick their opponents up when they got off the bus and wouldn't turn them loose until they were ready to go home.

Since the team didn't have any money for the tournament, they slept on the floor of the gym and ate out of a grocery store.

In the end they made the finals and lost by two to Jones High, the state champions. After that everybody wanted to know where under the sun that striped team had come from. And people were saying, "Don't you know? That's Little Elders's team."

That tournament made Oliver so well known that when Little Rock built a new black high school a few years later, the principal wanted Oliver as his basketball coach. When Oliver went up to interview, the two of them talked for a while about educational philosophy. At the end the principal asked him, "How'd you manage to beat Jones High in that tournament?" By that time everybody in Arkansas was remembering that little Almyra had actually won the game.

"We didn't beat them," Oliver said. "They won by two."

"Well," said the principal, "it was as good as beating them." Then he asked how fast Oliver could move up to Little Rock to coach his team.

———

I left for Minnesota in July. Originally my idea had been to complete my internship and pediatric residency there—that's three years. Then I would do a surgical residency—another two or three years—at which point I would be a full-fledged pediatric surgeon. But that was before Oliver. If I kept to that plan, it would mean Oliver having to move up to Minnesota. I didn't have any question that he would have done it. But it would have been a terrible wrench, tearing himself away from a career he loved in a place where he had gained a large reputation and everybody thought the world of him to go to frozen Minnesota and start over from nothing. I thought that wouldn't have just been senseless and unfair; it would have been cruel.

The result was that we didn't even really discuss it. I just made the decision to move back to Arkansas, where I knew Ted Panos was waiting to put me in as a pediatric resident. So after a year of interning in Minnesota, I came back. Ironically, I came back just as Oliver left to spend the summer semester at Indiana University, where he was enrolled in the graduate program in health and physical education. Indiana was a mecca for basketball, and Branch McCracken, the coach there, was the prophet of the fast break and the pressure defense, which was Oliver's game. Oliver's mother was one of those teachers who were totally devoted to their profession. She went to every professional conference she could make and never stopped experimenting with different ideas. That was the way Oliver was with his coaching. If Branch McCracken was giving courses somewhere, Oliver was going to be there.

While Oliver was away that summer, I went house hunting. I eventually found something I thought we'd both like in Glenview, a lower-middle-income black neighborhood in North Little Rock. It was a one-story brick house, with three bedrooms and one and a half baths. Small. But it had a nice lawn and plenty of room for a garden. Across the street was a big creek, and behind the house were a hundred acres of undeveloped land. I was awfully proud of that house.

That summer I planted lots of trees in the bare yard, and bushels of marigolds. Then I put in the garden: tomatoes and peppers and pole beans, lettuce, onions, radishes, watermelons, okra, and collards. This was my first house after years of living in dormitories and rented rooms and apartments. I was ready to bring some farm back in my life.

Being a resident at University Hospital was no joke. Residents taught and doctored. We worked in the clinic, conducted pediatric rounds, and supervised medical students and interns. Being on thirty-six hours straight was usual. You'd work all day, then all night, then all the next day. After that you could go home, but you'd be on call. That meant I was at the hospital every third night ordinarily, and likely as not I'd be in on other nights too. It was just plain brutal.

Everybody had a way of getting through. Mine was Oliver. He used to say he did his residency too, which is more or less true. Oliver would come over to the hospital the nights I was on duty so he could keep me company if I had some downtime. Sometimes he would come over and I'd be tied up with one emergency after another. But even then I made sure I saw him.

At midnight I'd grab a snack, and we'd go to the little resident's rest room and eat it together before I'd have to run back down to the emergency room.

Oliver's being there helped me get through the stress and the sleep deprivation. It was just comforting and somehow stabilizing to know he was going to be there. Like having a rock I could attach myself to. More than once I needed him a lot worse than he might have been completely aware of. My residency at Arkansas introduced me to some grim happenings, which I had a tendency to carry around with me.

The first of these was a thirteen-year-old girl who was referred to the hospital by her local physician not long after I arrived. Mary, a pretty little white girl from the Ozarks, was brought in by her mother. Her looks were distorted by a large goiter on her neck and bulging eyes, classic signs of hyperthyroidism. But there was more to the referral. Her doctor had also noted severe nervousness, smothering spells, high blood pressure, bed-wetting, weight loss, and poor performance in school.

We treated Mary for thyroid disease for almost two weeks at the hospital, and she did very well. By then she and I had become friends. When it seemed the problem was under control, I went in to tell her it was time to go home, which was something I always liked doing. Children were usually thrilled to death to hear they could go back to their families. But when I told Mary, she started crying. I sat down next to her on the bed, but at first she wouldn't say anything. She just didn't want to go.

After I had sat with her awhile, though, it came out. She said she hated Saturday nights. "Saturday nights my Daddy and my brother and my uncles use me," she said. I didn't know quite what she meant. She was weeping, and I wasn't sure I had heard her right.

"What do you mean, use you?" I said.

"They use me and my sister," she said. "Saturdays is when they get drunk. They take me and my sister out back, and they get on us."

I didn't know what to do, but I knew I needed to talk to someone. I thought about calling the police but decided to go first to the hospital social worker, Mr. White. Mr. White was a wonderful black man with a world of experience. "Dr. Elders," he said, "there's nothing we are going to be able to do about this. We can't prove what she's saying one way or another, so there's nothing to do but send her home. If you report this or bring charges or try to move her out of the house, they'll sue you. You're the one who will end up prosecuted."

This was five or six years before Arkansas changed its child abuse laws. I hadn't known anything about these situations because I had never dealt with one before. But I found out fast. No doctor ever reported suspected abuse back then. The best you could do was turn it over to your social worker, who would try to find a discreet way to talk to someone in the family. The whole legal and medical professions were working overtime to pretend this was a problem that didn't exist.

I still felt I couldn't just let this go and wash my hands. When Mary's mother came in, I got up my courage to talk to her, keeping in mind that I'd better not make any accusations. I told her I was concerned Mary might be being abused in some way. Did she possibly know of anything that could be going on, on Saturday nights, for instance? She said that some of them liked to go out and drink a little home brew on Saturdays and have a little fun. But they weren't doing anything where someone could get hurt. That was it. She said it, and there was nowhere else I could take it.

The end result was that we sent Mary home. But the worry stayed on my mind. I felt I had done something as a physician that I shouldn't have. She had escaped from that horrible den into my care for a few days. She had confided in me as a friend. And I had discharged her right back into it, without a doctor to follow her up and guide her and try to cure her real problem.

I saw Mary two more times over the next couple of months. Each time it was like opening a wound. Her thyroid problem was doing fine, but the last time I saw her it turned out she was pregnant. That was an additional shock, even if it wasn't exactly any surprise. I had grown up in a place where if you got pregnant as an unmarried teenager, your life was considered ruined.

It seemed very clear to me that Mary's life *was* ruined: a young girl with a baby fathered by one of her close relatives. But there was nothing to do about that either. Abortion was illegal at that time, period. Incest or not, it didn't matter. Ruined life or not. Today I think I would be pushing hard for an abortion in a case like this. Then it wasn't something I even thought about.

I think that was the first abuse case that left its mark on me. But after that I saw more than I bargained for, some sexual, more just physical. You'd know when a child was brought in with something broken and the mother would say he fell off the sofa. Here he's got a spiral fracture of the leg, which you just don't get from falling off a piece of furniture. But the parents would swear up and down that's what happened. So then you take whole-body X rays and you find there are old fractures and multiple fractures. Children fracture easily, but not that easily. Often it was from twisting arms. You see a spiral fracture on children, and you know without a doubt it was from parents twisting or jerking them.

You don't ease in gently with these kinds of things. They don't sit back and wait until you've matured as a doctor and developed ways of coping psychologically. The hardest thing I have seen in thirty-five years of medicine I saw as a young resident. It was a six-month-old baby who had been raped by a sixteen-year-old baby-sitter. She was torn and bleeding to death. To save her life, the surgeons had to go in and take out her uterus and cervix, then try to repair what was left. You bury sights like that somewhere inside of you. But if that's all you do with them, you will eventually find yourself in serious trouble. I'm not sure where my colleagues got their solace. I got mine from knowing that Oliver was there to latch on to.

You don't ease gently into death either. There was one indelible night my first year as a resident when I thought I would just have to give the whole thing up. That was a night I had five children die on my watch.

One of them was a six-year-old who had had surgery earlier that day. It wasn't something that anybody expected her to die of, but suddenly her heart stopped. I was working on this child feverishly. I had gotten an endotracheal tube in so she could breathe. Then I started pumping on her chest. When that wasn't working, the nurses had rushed in with the electrical defibrillators.

I was in the middle of jolting her with these when someone looked over at the other patient in the room, another six-year-old. She had been admitted with possible appendicitis, but the symptoms weren't clear, and we were watching her to see what might develop. Anyway, in the middle of all the commotion and urgency of trying to restart the one child's heart, one of the nurses looked at the other one and noticed that she wasn't breathing. I yelled at the medical student I had there to take over the defibrillators while I got a tube into the second one. Then we started cardiopulmonary resuscitation on her too.

By now all sorts of people were in the room, two other doctors, the nurses, medical students, a couple of aides. We had plenty of folks around to help, and I was doing everything I could think of and trying frantically to think of something else. But nothing was working. It was more and more desperate in there until we finally just got to the point where we had to accept that both these children were gone. And we didn't have any idea why. Neither one of them had had a good reason to die.

The first little girl had a congenital heart problem that the surgery was supposed to have taken care of. Either it hadn't, or there was some kind of unexpected postoperative shock. We never did find out about the second girl. The autopsy determined that her appendix was fine, but she had mesenteric lymphadenitis, enlarged lymph nodes in the abdomen, which can be painful but is not something you die of. We assumed the cause of death must have been some type of viral syndrome.

Not that it really mattered. I was still reeling from losing these two when I was called into the nursery to find that two very sick intensive care babies had just died. This wasn't the same kind of body blow as the first two. These were both tiny infants who had suffered brain hemorrhages and had sepsis. We were not expecting them to do well. But regardless, it's bitter to lose any child, let alone two at once. The parents of the first two were on their way into the hospital. I wasn't sure, but I thought that maybe the babies' parents were there already. I was just getting myself composed enough to go and look for them when a nurse came up to tell me that a little terminal leukemia girl we had on the floor had also just died.

There is no good way to tell parents the news of a child's death. As a resident I was still learning. I'm sure I'd still be learning today if I had much occasion to do it anymore. I like to go someplace quiet and sit down together; I think I knew that by then. Now I always make sure that the parents have an opportunity to see their child. You clean them up, get them ready, make sure there are clean sheets on the bed, so the parents can walk in with nobody else in the room and spend some time with their child. You give them the privacy to sit or talk or cry or whatever they feel they need to do. I feel that's so important. I learned that from personal experience when Oliver and I lost our last child in a stillborn birth and I wasn't going to be allowed to see him. I don't know if I understood that yet on that night when those five children died, but I may have.

The parents of the leukemia girl were distraught, even though they'd known she was in her last days. We all were distraught. By that time the staff was shell-shocked. We felt like we were walking through a battlefield full of corpses. But even with all their pain these parents were saying, "Oh, Dr. Elders, you did the best you could, you did the best you could." Here I was trying to reassure them, and they were the ones comforting me.

I didn't have the experience then. Now I know that the parents who are most demonstrative, the ones who fall out and scream and carry on, are very often the ones who have done the least for their children. There are other parents, whose pain you can see and feel, but somehow they are trying to comfort you; those are often the parents who have loved their children most deeply. That's true of white and black, rich and poor. Someone once asked me if over the years I have seen any differences in the emotional response of white and black parents. There is no difference. In the deaths of their children, parents just become parents. It's amazing how severe illness or death reduces us all to absolutely the same common human denominator.

Surgeons see the physical side of the common denominator every day of their working lives. Open a child up, and you can't tell what color he is. Under the scalpel it's all the same. But any doctor who works with parents comes to know that it's not just that we're alike physically. Dealing with suffering and death, you come to see that we are the same emotionally and spiritually as well.

It was about five o'clock that morning when I just lost it all. By then we had gotten everybody taken care of. All the children were down at the morgue. All the parents had gone home. That was when I got to sit down and write my reports about what had happened. I was sitting there at the desk with the two nurses, looking at the charts stuck up on the wall. They were writing up their notes, and I was writing mine when one of them turned to me and said, "It's been a tough night, Dr. Elders." That was just more than I could handle.

It was the only time in my career in medicine that I ever broke down and sobbed. The two nurses were in tears too, and they started hugging me and patting me and telling me it was going to be all right. "We'll go get you some coffee," they said. They wanted me to go sit in the conference room because I was right out there at the nurses' station in the hallway where patients or parents might come by, even though it was five o'clock and nobody seemed to be around but us.

But I didn't have the strength to move. At that moment it seemed to me that I was a failure, that I really just wasn't good enough. How could all these children have died and I couldn't do a thing about it? And then having to be so reassuring with the mothers and fathers. Talking death with the parents of those girls who had died in the room, then going right over to the babies' parents, then to the mother and father of the little leukemia patient. I felt shattered, like a piece of wreckage. I just didn't know if I could stand to do this anymore.

Chapter 8

Chief

❦

Thank God, that night was an aberration. We lost children. You do when you're handling severe birth defects and lots of referrals of especially difficult cases, which is what we got at the medical center. But I never experienced anything that bad again, and I never had quite that kind of reaction.

I was in my second year of residency when I started having my own babies. Oliver and I had planned it carefully. We wanted a family, and I was beginning to get on. In 1963 I was already twenty-nine, and in those days the word was that if you didn't have babies before you were thirty-three or thirty-five, you shouldn't be having them. That was considered about the outside without taking a significant risk of Down's syndrome or some other congenital defect. When our first son, Eric, was born, I looked at my chart, and the obstetrician had scrawled on it: "This old primagravita." I didn't know about that, but I probably was getting down toward the wire, especially considering we were planning to have several.

When I found out I was pregnant, I arranged my schedule so I could work up until my delivery date, which was what happened. The day Eric was born I was rounding all day on the pediatric wards. My back was hurting, so every once in a while I'd sit down and take a rest. Then I'd get up and go on to the next patient. At around five-thirty, when I was finished work I called Pat Reddin, who was the chief OB-GYN resident, and I told him that my back had really been bothering me all day. "Well," he said, "you'd better come down here and let me check you out before you go home."

I didn't think anything was really going on, but we lived in North Little Rock, which is easy to get to now, but wasn't until they built routes 630 and I-40. Now the drive takes fifteen minutes; back then it might have been thirty or forty. So I went down to maternity. When Pat took a look, he said, "Joycelyn, I don't think you better go home. I think we 'bout ready to have a baby." I was already several centimeters dilated.

By this time things were speeding up, and as I got into real labor, Pat said, "Okay, now I'm going to put in an epidural."

When he did, I lost feeling in the middle. I could tell when I was having contractions, and I could move my feet and hands and everything; I just didn't have any pain. "Heavens," I told him, "if it's this easy to have a baby, I could do it every day." I went in there at five-thirty, and at ten that night Eric was born.

There's probably some irony to this. All of us were born at home, and Mama tended to have difficult births. I was there for some of them, maybe most. I was out in the kitchen mainly, doing whatever Mother Sabie, the midwife, told me to do and listening to Mama yelling and screaming in the bedroom. I've heard that when I was born, she was so sick afterward she had to go stay with her mother, Elnora, for a month. She had developed what we would now call puerperal sepsis. Given the conditions, it's a wonder she didn't die of infection with either me or one of the others. Now there I was, having my first with an epidural and all the latest technology. Of course I worked up to the last minute too, like she always did, but it wasn't out in a field chopping cotton.

Oliver and I thought that Eric was the most wonderful, beautiful baby God had ever made. We were thrilled to death. I stayed home for six weeks, nursing him. Then I thought that if

I stayed home any longer, I just might not go back to work at all, which wasn't part of the plan we had figured out.

Mr. and Mrs. Harris, the older couple we stayed with after we were married, had never had their own children. They had more or less adopted Oliver in the time he lived with them; then they opened their arms to me after we got married. Even after we bought our own home, we stayed on close terms. So by the time Eric came along they felt they had grandparent status. They were eager to look after him however much we were willing to give him out.

I was torn about leaving Eric with anybody. But I had never seriously considered not working, and this was as close to a perfect solution to the baby care problem as we were going to get. Oliver was often out late with practices and ball games, and my schedule was its usual insanity. But Mrs. Harris was more family than she was a baby-sitter. We set up a whole nursery at her house and bought her a complete set of everything—diapers, equipment, formula. I washed my diapers, and she washed hers. I had my bottles, she had hers. We dropped Eric off with her in the morning and picked him up in the evening, except every third night when I was on call and Oliver came to the hospital to keep me company. Those nights Eric just stayed over.

I don't remember feeling guilty about leaving Eric. When we weren't at work, Oliver and I spent every moment with him. By the time he was two or three weeks old we were taking him to basketball games. If it was a home game, I'd pick him up at Mrs. Harris's on the way over. If it was away, we'd take him with us on the team bus. Whenever some crisis came up, I just brought him along to the hospital and put him to bed in the emergency room. While I was seeing about the patient, the nurses would keep an eye on him for me. The only thing I had a hard time adjusting to was losing my Sunday newspaper rights. In our pre-Eric days my one day off was Sunday, which I used to spend doing nothing except lie around drinking coffee and reading the paper. It was so luxurious getting up and getting the paper and a cup of coffee, then climbing back into bed. I loved everything about Eric, but it was probably years before I got to relax with that paper again.

———

When I finished my second year of residency, Dr. Panos asked me if I would consider being chief resident. "Joycelyn, we're going to have a real good crop of young doctors next year, and I think you'd make a real good chief resident. I talked to some of the other people and other services about it, and I talked to the dean about it, and I think I'd like to do that if you'd be interested. Why don't you give it some thought and come back and talk to me?" He'd always give you a time to come see him. "Why don't you think it over a few days? Come see me on Thursday, say, four o'clock."

Now this was a real honor. It was an unusual thing for a woman to be chief resident anywhere in those days, and for a black woman it was unheard of. But it wasn't just an honor because I was a black female in Arkansas. It was an honor because it was an honor. If Dr. Panos hadn't asked me, I wouldn't have thought about it one way or another. I wasn't expecting it in the first place, so I wouldn't have been hurt not getting it. But I wasn't really that surprised either. I had worked hard, and in my heart I thought I was the best-qualified resident on the pediatric service. If Panos and the others decided I was the right person to be chief, they wouldn't be getting any argument from me on it.

Of course I knew there might be a difficulty or two. As chief I would be head of nine other residents, all of them white southern males. I'd have to deal with all the other services about admissions and beds and the hundred problems and conflicts that came up every day, and no one would be too used to working on an even basis with someone like me. I'd also have to deal with doctors all over the state, and in some parts of Arkansas old-time attitudes hadn't changed. "Dr. Elders," a referring physician in the delta once told me about his patients—this was on the phone; we had never met—"Dr. Elders, don't you worry none about these people I'm sending you. They're just good ol' cotton patch niggers."

But the bottom line was that even if there was the potential for problems, I still didn't think there'd actually be any. I knew the service chiefs would keep their residents in line, if ever that was necessary, which was hardly likely. Some of the chiefs and senior faculty weren't as liberal as they wanted the world to think they were, but few of them were from either Arkansas or anyplace else in the South. Dr. Panos was from Wyoming, and Dr. Ebert was from Minnesota, and Dr. Schlumberger was from Ohio. Of course there was Dr. Brown, the OB-GYN chairman. He wasn't a liberal of any sort. He didn't think a black doctor could treat white women in Arkansas, at least not a black male doctor. That was a delicate subject for him. But of course that didn't exactly apply to me. I wasn't male and wasn't in gynecology. I was in pediatrics, and black women had been taking care of white children forever. So I didn't anticipate any problems even with him. I just didn't see any downside to this job. I was proud they had asked, and I was going to take it.

When I went back to Dr. Panos, we talked it over some more, and he told me again he thought I could handle it. He didn't say, "Joycelyn, I think you can handle it. But you should be aware of the concerns I have, and here they are." He just said I could handle it, and if ever I wanted to talk, I should think of him as my Dutch uncle and come see him. So with that blessing I became chief pediatric resident.

Now, I was sure there were things going on behind the scenes that I didn't know, and maybe I didn't want to know. Although I didn't let it concern me too much, there wasn't any doubt this was a groundbreaking move. It was only a few years back that Arkansas had become a national symbol of racism, with Orval Faubus facing off against President Eisenhower over the integration of Central High School. Of course that had shamed a lot of Arkansans. Race relations in the state weren't nearly as bad as they were being made out, and people didn't like their homeplace being thought of in those terms. But no question, there was a heavy racial backdrop to my appointment.

One of the people who knew things I didn't was Dr. Ed Hughes. Ed was a junior faculty member in both pediatrics and pathology, only about five or six years older than I was. He had trained in Utah and Minnesota, then had gone on to the Brookhaven National Laboratory. He was a salty westerner from some little place in New Mexico, a real home-on-the-range-type cowboy. But I thought he understood the physiology of medicine better than anybody I had ever met, and I still do to this day. He was maybe the brightest man around there, a really first-rate chemist and research scientist.

Ed and I had gotten to know each other well when I was a first-year resident. He was rounding with me in the nursery, and one of our cases there was a very sick baby who ended up precipitating my first real research. This baby had a markedly distended abdomen. She had obviously suffered some kind of catastrophic event, but we could not determine what it was, and we were struggling to keep her alive long enough so we could figure it out. We wanted to do an exploratory and kept pushing the surgeon on it. But he felt she was too sick to survive it and insisted he had to wait.

Ed and I worked really hard on that baby. For forty-two days we had IVs running into her giving her food and keeping her electrolytes just so, doing things that might look barbaric now but then were the only way we had of keeping her alive. In the process we learned a lot, especially about salt and water balance. But we never did find out what was wrong, and despite everything, we finally lost her.

I did the autopsy on this baby I had cared for so long, and we found she had a ruptured stomach. That was what she had died of. To have survived, she would have needed an operation probably within a day or two of the rupture, which of course hadn't been done because she was so fragile. What we didn't understand was, Why would a baby's stomach just spontaneously rupture? The stomach is a big, strong muscle, and an event like that is a rarity, which was the reason it hadn't occurred to us in all our worrying about the case.

So we started going through the whole list of things that could possibly make a stomach rupture. We set up experiments with mice and developed a device that could measure precisely how much pressure it took to rupture a mouse's stomach. We fed different groups of mice compounds—steroid hormones, salicylates, glucocorticoids, and so on—and we measured how much pressure it took to rupture the stomach. In the course of doing this we traced the mechanisms by which aspirin and steroids affect the stomach lining. To a certain extent the work enlarged our understanding of why people who are sensitive to steroids tend to get ulcers and how taking aspirin sometimes causes bleeding in the stomach.

We wrote our experiment up and published it as "Spontaneous Rupture of the Stomach: Clinical and Experimental Study." Though we didn't know for sure, we believed the baby's rupture was related to severe stress and increased amounts of glucocorticoids, similar to what happens with stress ulcers. These, we thought, weakened the stomach wall to the point that gaseous distension caused a tear.

Anyway, that was my introduction to Ed Hughes. He was one of Dr. Panos's young Turks, and he had an insider's view of events. Here's Ed's view of what went on, including the racial background I was doing my best to ignore. Ed: "Ted Panos initiated Joycelyn's appointment as chief resident. He was the son of a Greek immigrant, so maybe he had some minority feeling we didn't have. But he was still reluctant about it. He thought it would create a lot of turmoil, and things were still shaky politically. At one point old Faubus was going to shut down the medical school.

"See, we had gotten ourselves in a crack the year after Faubus closed Central High School. After that he closed down the whole public school system. In Little Rock there were no schools open for a year. But he didn't have the authority to do that himself. He had to get the school board to do it.

"Well, there was a recall law, and we were going to recall the entire school board that had done Faubus's bidding. We organized the STOP campaign, primarily out of the medical school. 'Stop This Outrageous Purge!' We were the instigators of that campaign; it was our thing. We had to get so many signatures. And that's all I did; I went door to door. It was amazing how easy it was to get people to sign. And we recalled that whole damned school board. That's when Faubus really got a hard-on for us.

"What he did was pull out all the welfare money we were running the hospital with. The state was feeding money to the medical school. We were a state hospital, so to speak. It was only about eight hundred thousand dollars a year, but then it was a lot of money. That was what we took care of the poor people with, and that was all we had—poor people. We had damned few paying patients with insurance. Ninety percent of our patients were poor. This was the 'nigger hospital,' although we had more poor whites than blacks. If you had money you went to one of the private hospitals, St. Vincent's, or Baptist, or Doctors'.

"Faubus pulled all the money out because he wanted us to collapse. To him we were a bunch of Communists and outsiders, and we were just down there causing trouble. Hell, we didn't go down there to save blacks or anything else. We went down there because we had chosen careers in academic medicine and we wanted a good pediatrics department. But with all this shit going on, how could you do that?

"Finally old Faubus backed down. He came out and had some meetings with faculty people. Ted took me to some of those. Our dean then was a very diplomatic guy, a typical proper Pennsylvania graduate. It was hard for him to bargain like we knew we were going to have to with a tough redneck like Orval Faubus. So Ted brought me along just to have another hard-shell western type with him. Eventually the Supreme Court found Faubus's faculty oath signing unconstitutional; he had made us all sign oaths that we weren't Communists. Then after that they found some reason why he had to restore the welfare money."

So that was the background. Now here's Ed on the actual appointment. "Ted sought our advice, and we sat around the table and thrashed it out. My contention was that all we had to decide was if Joycelyn was the best doctor we had on the resident staff. If we decided that, then she ought to be chief resident. I didn't give a damn if she was a woman. Of course being a woman was bad enough, but being a black woman? But it could be I wasn't too attuned. When I was applying to medical school in Utah up from New Mexico, the dean asked me in my interview, 'Mr. Hughes, what are we going to do about the Negro problem in the South?' I said, 'Well, Dr. Bauers, I don't know what we're gonna do with the Negro problem in the South. I never saw a Negro until I was about eight years old and I have no idea what the problem is.'

"Actually we knew how to discriminate in New Mexico pretty well. We had been doing it against the Spanish for a long time. But the thing that turned me into an integrationist was when one of Joycelyn's black classmates in medical school went to a football game in War Memorial Stadium and two burly state policemen came in there and hauled him out. Blacks weren't allowed in War Memorial Stadium. That's when I decided something's wrong down here. This ain't no way to treat hogs. William Mays is the one they dragged out. He was a fine young man who went on to become an internist in Michigan.

"I guess us white Anglo-Saxon son of a bitches are just sort of blind. When Joycelyn was in school, the black medical students couldn't eat with the white students. They had to go eat with the colored help in back of the kitchen. In retrospect, that was just awful. If that happened now, a hundred percent of the faculty would lose their minds. I know Ted was very upset by it. But he was politically savvy too. He knew how hard you could step. Now you look back on it, it sort of makes you feel guilty.

"But really, appointing Joycelyn wasn't a hard decision to make. There was no question she was the best we had. She was just a good doctor. She never gave up on a kid. She treated the mother too. The white mothers often liked Joycelyn better than they liked me, because she was so patient and understanding. Finally Ted decided he had to bite the bullet. I don't think he actually consulted the other chiefs. He was the kind of guy who ran his own ship. He was a typical Greek intellectual. If he thought it was right, he was going to do it.

"But before he actually appointed her, he sent Del Fisher and me out to kind of scout out the other residents and see what they'd say. Hell, they didn't care. They knew Joycelyn was headed for the top of the mountain."

I didn't know Dr. Panos had his staff talk to the residents, though I suspected that he had canvassed them in some way. But I knew them well myself, and I knew they were determined there were not going to be any black marks on Arkansas related to my being chief resident. They knew me too. I was sure they respected my competence as a doctor and my fairness. And they knew that I would protect their interests every way I could with the other services, that I'd tear into anybody for them.

From the moment I was appointed they treated me like they would have treated any chief. It was "Hi, Chief," from the first. It was almost as if they had gotten together and said, "We're going to be good. We've had enough trouble with Central High." But I think most important, they were a good group of young men whose hearts were in the right place. A few of those guys are still around Little Rock, and when I see them today they still call me Chief. Sam Boellner, who's the neurologist here, was one of them. So were Dale Briggs and Jerry Jones, who are pediatricians at Children's Hospital. Sam was probably the person who influenced the thinking of that group most. He had been the top student in his class at the university medical school, then had gone off to Vanderbilt to do an internship before coming back for his residency. I've always felt very good about Sam because I believe he could have broken me that year if he had wanted. He was the most senior resident, he was extremely bright, and he was from a very influential family here in town. He really had the capacity. But he used it to make sure things went smoothly.

That year was without a doubt the hardest year of my life. I worked 365 days. I made rounds every single day and was responsible for every pediatric admission. There was more than one time when parents were surprised to find themselves dealing with a black physician. Every once in a while I'd have a parent actually tell me, "Dr. Elders, my doctor told me to come in and see you, but I didn't want to come. I asked him was there someone else I could go to and he said no." But the bottom line was that if their child was sick and their doctor had told them I was the best one to take care of it, they came. And when you're successful, parents think you are not just good, you are supergood. They think you are better than you are. When you heal somebody's child, you are at the right hand of God.

I'm writing this now in August 1995, thirty two-years after Ted Panos appointed me chief. This has been a hard time for Oliver and me because our second son, Kevin, is appealing his conviction on a drug offense. Yesterday I was sitting at Kevin's trial, and there was an older couple in the courtroom whom I didn't know. They were white, and they were sitting there with no one else but us and the judge and lawyers. At one of the breaks the woman came up to me and said, "Oh, Dr. Elders, I just came to offer you my support. I know you don't remember me, but you saved my child. We've always been grateful, and we've been behind you." And I have people from twenty-five and thirty years ago, back to when I was a resident even, who still come up and tell me something I did for their child. Most of the time I don't remember, unless maybe it was an unusual endocrine case. But that's of no importance. They say what's in their hearts. And whether or not I was who they expected me to be when they first brought their child in doesn't make any more difference to them than it ever did to me.

Chapter 9

Wasting Disease

❧❦❧

"I'm going into practice." That's what I told Ed Hughes at the end of my year as chief resident when he asked what I was planning to do.

"Oh, you're a damned liar," he said. "You don't need to go out and practice, you wouldn't be worth a damn in practice. We need some black doctors on the faculty. Why don't you go into research so you can learn to be a decent faculty person?"

I didn't know until I started digging into the past for this book that Ted Panos had put Ed up to this little tirade. Until he said it, I wasn't feeling any great tug to go into academic medicine. To the contrary, I had probably spent more time being trained as a clinical pediatrician than almost anybody: my internship at Minnesota, then a straight two-year residency, plus the chief residency. That was four years of pediatric training when three was more usual. Although I liked experimental work, I hadn't felt a big compulsion to go into research either. More than anything, I thought of myself as a baby doctor.

"Well," I said, "I can go and be a decent faculty person and work in the clinics."

"Aw, hell," Ed growled, "you can't work in no clinics. You won't ever get promoted. Besides, you already know about doctoring. What you've got to learn now is more biochemistry because you don't know a damned thing about that."

The more I thought about it, the more the idea made sense, especially considering Eric, and Oliver's and my plans to have more children. If I were in practice, I'd have no control over my life. My time would belong to my patients, not me. But if I did research, I could work all day and night if I wanted, Saturdays and Sundays too. But I would be the one who controlled it. That way I could combine being a mother and a doctor on my own terms.

Oliver also thought academic medicine had a lot of pluses and agreed that's what I should try for. When I went back to Ed, he suggested the way to do what we wanted was for me to apply for a National Institutes of Health (NIH) three-year fellowship grant with him serving as my sponsor. If we got that, the award would pay for my salary as a researcher and junior faculty member. At the same time I could work for a doctorate in biochemistry. Well, I liked chemistry, but I didn't think I liked it a Ph.D.'s worth, especially not after being in school and training almost more years than I could count. But by the time Ed and I finished kicking and scratching about it we had agreed that at least I'd do a master's.

One thing I knew for sure while we were planning out our NIH grant proposal: I knew it was unusual for a smart, upcoming young male professor to take a black woman on as a fellow. I mean, male professors weren't even interested in women, let alone blacks. Blacks and women were just kind of over there in a pile; they didn't worry about them. What they wanted to have as a fellow was a bright young white man just like themselves. I knew that with Ed Hughes I hadn't found just a sponsor; I had found a mentor.

I was equally lucky having Ted Panos as my department head. Dr. Panos was a wonderful, wonderful person, even if in some ways he was also a man of his time. Despite his basic fairness, he held firm to a couple of old-fashioned ideas. One of these was that women doctors didn't deserve to make as much money as men. It wasn't that he believed women shouldn't be doctors or they shouldn't have a chance at advancement. He had a lot of women in his department then and later—Rosalind Abernathy, Vida Gordon, Lee Berry, Florence Char, and Alice Beard, as well as myself—but he didn't think they should be paid equally. He seemed to believe their husbands ought to be supporting them. That kind of double standard was a sore point, but there was no question we all owed a huge debt to Ted.

———

The research we proposed, and the NIH approved, was on the function of the thymus gland in newborn mice. What precipitated my interest in this was a particular deadly syndrome we saw in human newborns called wasting disease. For some unknown reason certain infants would not grow but instead lost weight, withered, and soon died despite all our efforts to keep them alive. Once the syndrome set in, it was invariably fatal. This wasting disease was a mystery; no one had any idea why it happened. Like many pediatricians, I had racked my brains over the puzzle without getting anywhere.

At just about this time Dr. Robert Good at the University of Minnesota discovered that the thymus gland has an important effect on the immunological system. Among other things, he noticed that if he removed the thymus from newborn mice, they developed what looked like the same wasting syndrome we were seeing in babies. Good was probably the world's leading pediatric immunologist; his discoveries eventually won him the Lasker Prize in medicine, the so-called American Nobel. I had known him well when I was at Minnesota as an intern and was familiar with his work, which was what led me to the research we had proposed.

I was studying the effect of thymus removal on mice, trying to track down exactly why it led to wasting disease, when we noticed something unusual. I say "we," but it was really Bernice Parham, the lab assistant who took care of the mice and actually performed the thymectomies. "This may not be any of my business," she said one day, "but you know, the females that are pregnant don't get wasting disease."

When I started looking at that, I discovered that the infants of thymectomized females had developed abnormally large thymus glands. And it was true, the thymectomized mothers didn't get wasting disease. On the other hand, when the pregnancy was completed, they did develop the disease. When we examined the biological role of thymic hormones, we found that the thymuses of the fetal mice were feeding the hormone to their thymectomized mothers.

Our discoveries in this area led to a broader understanding of the role the thymus plays in the body's immunological system. Subsequent research, which built on our findings, established that one of the functions of the thymus is to make immune cells competent. Lymphocytes that are processed through the thymus learn to identify specific bacteria and viruses so they can attack them. All these lymphocytes' daughter cells will "inherit" the information. They too will be able to identify and attack. But if the thymus is removed, the lymphocytes are unable to tell enemy from friend. The immune system won't work. In effect, removing the thymus produces an artificial AIDS.

At the same time we were looking at mouse thymus glands, we had other studies going on in the lab, including research on the metabolism of bone growth. For a while I was up to my ears in lab chickens, which we were using for this study, and I guess I was thinking and talking about chickens more than people commonly do. One time, when I was visiting home, my father finally got exasperated with it. "You know," he snapped at Mama, "she says she's a doctor. But all she ever talks about is chickens. I thought she knew what to do with chickens before she left from down here."

Ed Hughes had done some of the early studies on how growth hormones work, and he was a bulldog at tracking these things down. He never let go of a problem once he had his teeth in it, and he never just accepted some explanation because that was the way people always understood it. "Well, goddammit, why?" he'd say. As much of a cowboy roughneck as he was, it always amazed me how plain smart he could be and what a profound knowledge he had of organic chemistry.

While we were doing this, I was also taking biochemistry courses at the university. I got so involved trying to understand the biochemical basis of disease and deficiencies that I ended up doing forty-six class units more than I needed for a master's degree. The other side was that even though we were turning out numerous articles on our research, I found it really frustrating trying to sit down and write up my main work as a formal thesis. It just didn't seem to want to go, and I thought I was too busy and spread thin to take the time to make it. According to Ed, he practically had to throw me in the Arkansas River to make me do it.

That's not far from the truth; it *was* like pulling teeth. When I finally did write the thing, I gave it to him and Del Fisher to critique, and they just chopped it to bits. Ed tells me I was so mad I threw it back down on his desk and announced that if he didn't like the damned thing, I didn't either and I wasn't going to finish it. "All right," he said. I remember this clearly because he was so quiet and rational instead of ratcheting up the volume. "All right, so you won't get a master's degree—even though you've done all this work for it. But you know, Joycelyn, if you're going to make it in this racket, you're going to have to be able to put things down on paper so they're acceptable." I stewed over that for a couple of weeks. Then I sat down and did a complete revision.

The fact is that I had a lot of distractions going on in my life at that point, one of them being the birth of our second son, Kevin. Finishing the thesis right then just didn't seem like that big a priority.

Kevin was due on August 21; this was in 1965. It so happened that the final exam for the statistics course I was taking was on August 21. But several days before that I began feeling I was getting ready to have this child. I was thinking, Please, please don't let me deliver this one until I'm finished with my test. I was gritting my teeth and holding on, even though I knew without a shred of doubt that if he was ready to come, he was going to come. By the time I sat down to take that exam I was fit to be tied. I thought, Okay, if I make it through this, I'm getting someone to carry me straight down to the delivery room, and if they're not ready for me over there, God help them.

To my great surprise, Kevin let me finish that test. Then, despite lots of false starts and commotion, I didn't go into real labor until the twenty-sixth, which was when he finally got himself born. That was the longest six days I have ever lived or ever hope to live. I felt I had been in labor for a month.

———

Kevin's arrival meant some rearrangement in our lives. First of all, we had to find someone to take care of him during the day. Also, Eric was almost three now, which meant he was running all over the place and getting to be a handful for the Harrises. For some time we had been thinking about getting Eric into some kind of social and learning situation where he could be with other children.

In the reading Oliver and I were doing about early-childhood education we had come across Maria Montessori. She had ideas about children's creativity and their innate drive to learn that really made sense to both of us. Plus, she talked about how ages three to six represent a special period of potential, which of course caught our attention.

There weren't any Montessori schools in Little Rock we could go and look at, but there were other people around who were interested in her ideas. At that time I was a member of something called the Panel of American Women. This was a national organization that presented talks and discussions by women on social issues, mainly the experiences of blacks and whites with each other and the prospects for integration. Some of the people I knew from the panel had young children, and they were talking about Montessori too. Finally we decided to look into setting up a Montessori school ourselves.

As we got serious about this, one of the women suggested that we invite someone from the Montessori movement to come and talk to us. We did that, and shortly afterward we took a deep breath and decided to go ahead with it. The Montessori movement sent us two teachers from Germany, a husband and wife, we found a place to rent, and soon we had a going school.

Meantime Oliver and I had hired a woman, Mrs. Williams, to come and take care of Kevin and Eric at our house. When the Montessori school finally opened up, we would take Erie there in the morning on our way to work. Since Oliver couldn't leave school easily, I'd go and pick Eric up at twelve o'clock when the half-day session was over, drop him home, then drive back to the hospital.

This wasn't an ideal situation, but it was the best we could manage. I was agitating some for the medical school to provide day care, along with Barbara Kilgore and Loretta McNatt, two research assistants in Ed Hughes's lab. With all the hours we spent together, Barbara and Loretta and I were becoming close friends. Later on I think Ed began to regard us as a kind of hotbed of feminism, which was probably an exaggeration. But we never did stop trying to get the medical school to set up day care. We never got it either. "Can't imagine why not," Ed would chortle. "All it is is space and money."

Before Kevin, Oliver and I spent all the time we could with Eric. Now that Kevin had arrived we found we were practically hermits. Our social lives consisted of going to basketball games and being with the boys. On Saturdays and Sundays I'd pack up a picnic and the stroller and we'd go out to Burns Park in North Little Rock, where there were lots of activities for children—swings and miniature trains and a little petting zoo. People at the medical school used to wonder why I was never at the faculty cocktail parties and other social events. Ed Hughes couldn't have cared less. But some of the others did, and I'd often get these pointed "Why weren't you there last night? Where were you?"—type questions.

I always made some lame excuse. It wasn't that easy just to say, "Well, Professor, I was spending the time with my family." The fact is, I would have had a hard time going to those parties even if we hadn't been busy with Eric and Kevin. I was always uncomfortable in situations like that. I wasn't very good at making small talk, and I didn't especially like the kind of gossip you tended to hear at those things. I always thought I was really friendly, but I knew I didn't have any idea how to be a party person. Oliver was even worse than I was. Unlike me, he was kind of shy to begin with. I think he'd rather be boiled in oil than have to spend an evening drinking and smiling at people he didn't know. Besides, now that I didn't need to be on call anymore I found I was going back to keeping the kind of hours I had grown up with on the farm—in bed early and up before daybreak.

———

Eight or nine months after Kevin was born I began to notice that Oliver seemed to be going through a bad period at school. He was ordinarily on the quiet side with other people anyway, even though he and I talked to each other all the time. But now he seemed even quieter, and we weren't discussing things between ourselves nearly as much. I wasn't all that sensitive to it at first. Between the boys and work and keeping the house going, I know I was not paying as much attention as I should have been. Then one day Oliver came home from school obviously upset about something.

I was in the kitchen trying to cook supper and feed the baby and two or three other things, and Oliver was saying, "Sug, something happened to me today, and I'm really upset and I need to talk to you."

And I was saying, "Well, Sug, why don't you sit down awhile?" basically telling him he had to wait until I got through with supper and whatever else.

Suddenly he exploded at me. That was so un-Oliver. It was the last thing in the world Oliver would ever do. That was when I knew something was really wrong.

After that, it was as if he began shutting down. He talked less and less and lost interest in things that were going on in our lives. It seemed like he was withdrawing into some kind of shell. I didn't know what to do. Practically from the moment we met, Oliver had been my very best friend. He was the one

I went to when I had problems; in fact it was Oliver who kept me from having problems in the first place. I had long ago gotten dependent on him to be my rock. And now I couldn't *talk* to him anymore. Plus I had these two babies. After a while I began feeling like the world was closing in on me as well as him. I started feeling a little scared.

I thought, Maybe it's me or the boys. But there was no way of telling. He got more and more withdrawn until he was saying nothing at all. The weather was warming up into a typical late spring in Arkansas, and he would just go out into the backyard and sit there in the heat. In June he was going to have to go off to Indiana for the summer semester; he was still taking graduate classes for his athletic director's degree. I thought that maybe when he got there, it would be better. He'd be away from us and surrounded by talk about basketball and coaching. But when he went up there, things got worse, not better. I had to drive up to Bloomington and bring him home.

When he got back, I understood we were in serious trouble. That whole summer after I brought him home he just sat out back in the chair with his jacket on in the 105-degree sun. He didn't say a word. He just sat there, almost catatonic, in a profound depression.

I don't know how, but somehow Oliver managed to get himself to work when the school year began. But if anything, his state of mind was even more desperate. I'd get calls from him— "Sug, I'm dying"—and he'd race over to my office so I could look at him. I'd put the stethoscope on his chest and listen to his heart pounding away, knowing he was having a panic attack.

"It's all right," I'd say, "it's all right, Sug," knowing it wasn't and feeling my own heart pounding almost as hard as his was.

The psychiatrist we started going to together was trying to get to the bottom of the problem, but I couldn't see that we were making much progress. Basketball season arrived, a time when Oliver was always in his element. But it soon got to the point where he was too agitated even to sit on the bench with his team. "Get a walkie-talkie," I told him. "You can call the plays from up in the stands," I said, trying to sound as if this were somehow normal: the best basketball coach in Arkansas talking to his assistant on a walkie-talkie.

He actually tried that for a while, and his assistant, U. S. Grant, listened and relayed what Oliver told him. U. S. Grant was a wonderful young man who seemed to understand something about what Oliver was going through and tolerated all the strangeness without being anything but helpful. Sitting up in the stands next to Oliver, I watched what was happening, and I was swept by feelings of thankfulness, to him and to the team captain, Larry Lowe. Writing this, I couldn't remember his name at first and had to ask Oliver. But I will never forget that boy. All season he kept the players in line. They would get emotional and loud about something, and he could see Oliver getting upset and he'd just stop it. He'd get everything back in order. He was a young man with understanding beyond his years and the strength to lead those others. He stood very tall that season.

At one point Oliver's principal called me wanting to know what was going on with him. He knew something was wrong, he said, and he wanted to help if he could. He started giving Oliver flexibility, allowing him to leave school if he thought he had to or to take time for himself. Oliver had sympathetic people all around him, but none of it was doing any good, either for him or for me. Things finally got so bad that I didn't feel I could bear it anymore. I even began wondering if maybe the only way out of this might not be to kill myself. I caught myself having suicidal thoughts, especially when I was driving alone in the car. It seemed like it would be such an easy thing to do.

Finally the psychiatrist told me he thought my problems had gotten to the point where I needed a doctor too. He couldn't be my doctor because he was Oliver's, but he could recommend some people. One was the chairman of psychiatry, whom I started seeing every week. I had never in a million years imagined I'd end up in this situation. I still couldn't believe it. How could this be me all this was happening to? But I had to admit it was.

I tried whatever I could think of that might help. I thought, if only he could relax and get his mind off whatever fears he had that were doing this to him. Oliver had never had a lot of social kinds of friends. But I was constantly trying to get the ones he did have, and mine too, to take him fishing or do something else with him. Some of them did try, but he wouldn't go. He *would* go with me to church, but it was almost impossible for him to sit through the service. He'd get so agitated he'd be on the verge of getting up to leave. Then he'd grab my hand and clench it hard until service was over.

Oliver was in such despair that he wanted to go into a hospital. But his doctor wouldn't let him and insisted he keep coming to see him as an outpatient. That could have been a positive sign—maybe he thought Oliver wasn't sick enough for confinement—or maybe it was negative, that a hospital wouldn't do any good anyhow. I couldn't tell. By that time I couldn't tell much. I had hunkered down into the narrowest sphere I could. I took care of the boys, and I went to the lab. Beyond that someone else was going to have to do it; it was all I could do to try to hold me together.

I often wonder, Would I have coped if I hadn't had the friends I did? I found my solace in Barbara and Loretta at the lab and in Portia Powers, my friend who lived across the way. At home, whenever I felt myself unraveling, I'd run over to Portia's and blurt out, "Portia, I can't take it another day. I just can't make it." She'd say, "Yes, you can, Joycelyn. You can. You can make it another day and the next day too."

When I came home from work, I'd go over there just to talk to her for a few minutes, to calm down and gather my strength before stepping into my own house.

I hated weekends, when I had to be home. Friday afternoons were the worst; they filled me with dread. But I loved Mondays. The lab was a haven of peace and sanity. Barbara and Loretta, the research assistants there, were both a little younger than I was and both married with children. The exciting part of research is designing the experiments. Actually gathering the data can be tedious work, depending on what you are doing. A major focus of my research at that point was bone growth, which involved gathering chicken cartilage for analysis, a job we had started calling pickin' chickens. It wasn't the kind of work that required your full, concentrated attention. We picked chickens at the lab table and talked for hours on end, days on end, about everything under the sun: our children, their friends, our husbands, our hopes, our lives.

The love and support I got at the lab helped keep me abovewater. But it didn't do anything to solve my problems. As time went on, I began sorting things out. The conviction began growing on me that my main obligation was to take care of Eric and Kevin and raise them. To do that, though, the first thing was that I had to survive myself. To do that, I was going to have to separate myself from Oliver. At some point it dawned on me: I was going to have to leave. I needed to get a divorce.

I didn't feel I had a choice. That was the only way I could think of to save my life. I just could not stay there forever, I didn't have the strength for it. But I also knew I couldn't possibly leave Oliver while he was so desperately ill. Finally I decided that I would just wait until he got a little bit better. As soon as I saw even a slight improvement, I was going to take the boys and get out of there.

On my next visit to my psychiatrist I told him what I had decided. The moment Oliver was a little healthier, I was going to leave. All I wanted was for him to get well enough so that I could divorce him. He looked at me. This was the chairman of the department; he had seen the case records. "Joycelyn," he said, "Oliver is never going to get better."

Chapter 10

Arkansas's Expert

❧❦❧

When I heard this, my own instinct for survival started kicking in for real. If I couldn't divorce Oliver, I was still going to have to get away from him somehow, and the only way I could think to do that now was by pulling even further inside the cocoon I had woven around myself and the boys. I was so withdrawn that it took me awhile to realize that the medication Oliver was taking must have started having some kind of effect.

It wasn't anything major, just enough so I eventually took notice. One Sunday afternoon, when we got home from another endless church service, I asked, "You want to go out to the park?" It was just a mechanical question. I didn't expect anything. By now I never expected anything except either silence or agitation. But this time, instead of not answering, Oliver said softly, "Well, if you want to." After that every Sunday right after church I packed up a picnic and we went out with the boys. To someone else it might have seemed like a nice family outing. You probably couldn't have told from looking that Oliver was suffering the tortures of the damned, except a little numbed out now by the drugs, or that I was watching his every movement and trying not to be so distracted that I forgot about the boys.

Still, after a while we got to the point where Oliver and I could take a walk together, or maybe even go someplace to eat, just us, without Eric and Kevin. Nothing magic ever happened. But slowly, over months, so gradually I could never even tell if one day was truly better than the last, Oliver started talking again. Every once in a while he'd even say something on his own, not just some one-word answer to a question, but almost like he was trying to initiate something.

During this whole period I was doing my best to keep Eric and Kevin quiet, so as not to upset Oliver, which was no easy job considering their ages. I was constantly on edge about that. Keeping hushed up didn't come any more naturally to me than it did to either of them. It was a sign of how desperate I was that I had all of us walking on eggshells. This whole time Oliver's psychiatrist kept telling me, "Why do you tolerate that? Why do you accept him acting like that? Why don't you tell him that he can't act that way?"

I don't know if it had anything to do with this advice, but one day we all were tiptoeing around the house and I was getting so worked up that I just didn't think I was going to be able to stand it another second. I can't begin to remember what it was about, something of no significance, a glass of water or something. But whatever it was, I just blew my top at him. I started screaming at the top of my lungs. I bet I did that for thirty minutes straight. Every time he'd start trying to say something, I'd scream, "You just shut up!"

"But, Sug—"

"You just shut up. You just shut up and listen to me!"

And I got on with it. I just let everything out, a year or a year and a half's worth of frustration and anger at Oliver for being sick like he was. I know he had never heard anything like that out of my mouth before.

When I finally wore myself down and was out of breath, he looked at me and started to laugh. "Hey," he said, "you were really mad, weren't you?"

I was amazed. That was the most he had said for longer than I could remember. I said, "Yes, I was."

And he said, "Well, you sure sounded like it." Then he started laughing again.

That was the first healthy thing I had seen Oliver do since he had fallen into this depression. After that it just slowly started getting easier. Among other things, I began to do what the psychiatrists were telling me. When Oliver did something I didn't like, like sitting there as if he were comatose while I was talking to him, I'd say, "Listen, I am not going to sit up here and talk to you and you not answer me. If you're having a hard time hearing me, just say so. If you don't want to listen to me, just say so! But don't you sit there and not say anything to me while I'm talking to you, you hear me?"

I got very aggressive and demanding, so much so that sometimes I hardly recognized myself. When I thought about it, it seemed to me that what I was really saying with these outbursts was that I thought he was better, that he was all right now, and since he was, he had to start acting like a normal person, whereas before, when I was creeping around the house like a burglar, trying to keep myself and everyone else hushed up, it probably looked to him as if I were accepting the things he was doing. He knew that was not me. And if I wasn't being myself, it must have been because I thought that something was very badly wrong with him.

———

I felt so fragile myself that I hardly trusted my perceptions anymore, but slowly our lives seemed to be getting back to something like what they were before. To this day I do not know where Oliver found the resources to battle like he did, but as time passed, it was undeniable that he really was dragging himself back from the brink.

While Oliver was regathering his strength, I was getting near the end of my three-year fellowship and talking to Ed Hughes about what to do next. The upshot was that I applied for an NIH career development award, again with his sponsorship. These development awards provided support for five years to young doctors who wanted to make careers in research and whose work looked promising. Competition for them was fierce. But having had an NIH fellowship already, I was at an advantage. The NIH tended to think of career grants as a natural follow-up. They had already paid for training you for three years, and you had a track record with them. So if they were happy with that, it made sense for the NIH to continue to support you into the next phase of your career. The grant paid your salary, so that you were free to your medical school while you learned to develop your research skills and become a good teacher.

When I received this award, it was a coup in a way, not just for me but for Ed Hughes and Ted Panos, especially when an additional research grant came through that gave me enough funding to set up a laboratory. But I can't say I gave it all that much thought at the time. I had been working for the NIH for the last three years, and now I was still working for them. Life just seemed to be continuing on, with teaching and work in the lab and Oliver and the boys at home. But at the same time this new grant pretty much solidified my position as a faculty member and as someone whose research was being recognized.

The real excitement of being in this position hit home when I was invited to give a paper to the annual meeting of the Society for Pediatric Research. This was more than just exciting; it was enough to scare your hair white. The society was one of the world's most prestigious pediatric organizations. Its yearly meeting always attracted two thousand or so of the top medical scientists in the field. According to Ted Panos, nobody from the Arkansas medical school had ever been invited to address the plenary session before. He and Ed Hughes and Del Fisher were as proud as could be. I think they were also even more nervous about it than I was.

With something this big, they weren't about to be taking any chances. My presentation was going to be on the thymus research we had done on mice, showing the relationship between thymic hormone and wasting disease. Those had been my experiments, and along with Ed Hughes, I knew more about this subject than anyone. Ted wanted to make absolutely sure this presentation was going to go perfectly.

To him, as an old classics student who was devoted to the king's English, that meant getting rid of all the leftover country elements in my speech, which meant practice. After I wrote up my presentation, that man must have made me practice it a thousand times, which doesn't seem to me like much of an exaggeration. I gave that talk to him in his office time after time, listening to him correct this or that. Then I'd give it again. When I had finally gotten everything perfect enough for his satisfaction, he and Hughes and Del Fisher made me give it in the big auditorium, so that I'd have an idea of what was required in order to project sufficiently. They sat back at the other end, and I boomed it out until they were satisfied that every word was clear and crisp.

That paper on thymic hormone may have been the most practiced scientific presentation that has ever been given in the history of scientific presentations. I could have given it in my sleep. In fact I was giving it in my sleep. For days before the society's meeting I was dreaming about it. I could recite that thing at the push of a button, polished and clear as a bell and as loud as two thousand pediatric researchers could possibly want it.

When I finally did stand up in front of that crowd in Atlantic City's Steel Pier Convention Center, it was almost an anticlimax. The slides showed the normal thymus of a neonatal mouse next to the hugely enlarged thymus of an infant whose mother had been thymectomized. They looked like two silver dewdrops on a black background. They were so beautiful that textbook editors started clamoring after Ed Hughes and me for the rights to reproduce them.

The speech itself went perfectly. Afterward people told me they thought it was the best-delivered scientific presentation they had ever heard, which of course it should have been, given the amount of practice that went into it. The only tense moment was when one famous scientist, who was well known for his argumentativeness and ornery criticism of just about everything, got up and asked me to speculate on my findings. When he said that, I just knew that Ted and Del and Ed were holding their breath and right on the edge of having themselves coronaries. I had practiced the delivery until I was blue in the face, but speculation was something else altogether. I was still a fellow. What did I know about speculating, especially in front of this crowd? Two thousand senior scientists were sitting there, and there wasn't so much as a cough. "Well, Doctor," I said, giving it my best enunciation, "I am quite sure your own speculations on this subject are far more valuable than mine could ever be." Then I smiled at him. There was a long moment of silence; then a roar of laughter went up that filled the hall and drowned out the deep sighs of relief that must have been coming out of the Arkansas section.

———

I gave that presentation in 1967. I was thirty-four years old then and closing in on the outside limit of safe childbearing as it was believed in those days. Oliver and I had wanted at least three, but during his illness another pregnancy was the last thing on my mind. As he recovered, though, we began to talk about it, and we finally decided it was time. So early that year I got pregnant.

As usual, I went on working right up to my delivery date. Also as usual, between the clinic and the laboratory and teaching, I was running around so much I hardly had a moment to think. I didn't have any problems with the pregnancy, and as I got near term, I was as comfortable carrying this child as you can be after nine months of it. But on the Sunday before he was due I suddenly became aware that I couldn't feel any movement. I poked and poked and still couldn't get any response. When I called the doctor, he told me to come in immediately for an ultrasound, which back then was used only in certain unusual situations.

After examining me carefully, the doctor said he thought he could hear a heartbeat. Things sounded as if they were okay. That was reassuring, even though I still couldn't feel anything.

But over the next day or two I got more and more anxious. I could just tell there was nothing going on. When I called again, they had me come in for an X ray. By then I already knew what they were going to find.

This time it took the obstetrician only a couple of minutes before he told me he was going to put me out and induce labor. The last thing I remember was the anesthesiologist holding my hand and asking me to count. When I woke up much later and finally got my bearings, I couldn't recall anything that had happened. Then I heard the doctor telling me that the baby had been stillborn. It had been a boy, seven pounds, ten ounces. He had died, they said, from the umbilical cord having gotten wrapped around his neck. The obstetrician thought the baby had been dead for at least several days.

When I asked to see the baby, I was told I couldn't. But I just felt I needed so badly to see him. I had carried this child for nine months, feeling him growing and moving and imagining what he was going to be like. But when he was delivered, I wasn't even there. I was gone out to wherever the sodium pentothal had put me. I had no actual memory of him, of what he looked like and had grown into. All I was left with was the feeling of having had him inside me. I don't know why exactly, but it just seemed absolutely necessary for me actually, physically to see him.

Everyone was saying I couldn't, so from my bed I called J.D., the man in charge of the hospital morgue. The morgue staff knew me down there. I had taken my rotation in pathology and had done many autopsies myself. "I need to see him," I told J.D.

He may have understood. At least he wanted to help me out. "All right, Dr. Elders," he said. "I'll arrange it. I'll have everything set up for you."

When the nurses finally saw that I was going to get myself down to the morgue one way or another, they put me in a wheelchair and pushed me. Then they left me alone with him. I had done this same thing more times than I wanted to recall with parents who had lost children. I don't think this was something I had learned from anyone. It had always just seemed to me that the mothers and fathers should have a moment by themselves to say their good-byes. It had never occurred to me that one day I would be down here doing it myself.

Seeing that child then and thinking about him after, I was not conscious of my mother's presence. But I think her spirit was there, or at least her faith. When I looked to God on this, I did not expect to find any answers, no more than Mama expected to find them when her life had been stricken by some calamity. I have never believed that because of my prayers, God was going to give me this or that—either the answers I'd like to have or anything else. And somehow I have never quite felt I needed to go begging Him. But I did search my heart for how best to accept what had happened.

I always say that I feel my God will take care of me, and I believe He has, even if at times in my life it has not been immediately clear to me how. But with this child, from the moment I woke up from anesthesia and was told, I felt a great inner sense of relief. I can't say how long it had been before I was aware that his movement had stopped. But when I went in for the ultrasound that Sunday, it had been some time already. They could have done a C-section right then. I don't know what might have happened if they had. But by the time they did induce labor, there was no doubt the baby had been deprived of oxygen for a long, long time. His brain had suffered irreversible trauma. Had he lived, there is no question at all that he would have been severely handicapped. I had seen and treated so many terribly damaged babies. I knew exactly what kind of devastation that meant for them and for their parents.

There in that bed I said to myself, He's died, and that's best. I was not sure then, and I don't know now, that I would have been a good mother for a child who was severely mentally retarded. I know myself well enough to understand that I probably would have been greatly overprotective, even to the extent of neglecting the rest of my family to take care of him. I had seen that exact thing time and again when I was in medical school and working summers as a physical therapist at a camp for handicapped children in Massachusetts. More than a few of the parents who brought their sons and daughters with cerebral palsy and Down's syndrome and multiple handicaps there adored their children and were consumed by their problems.

Knowing my own emotions and my tendencies, I could just see myself in some of them. And though I can't say for sure, I feel that I would've been there, trying to make him get up to where he might have been, that I would have devoted my whole life to doing that. God knew, I thought, that I would not make a good mother to that child, that it would have put too great a burden on me and kept me from taking care of the others who needed me. I think He let it rest at that.

———

Working on the NIH career development grant with Ed Hughes as my mentor, I was becoming an experienced biochemistry-metabolism person. But in Arkansas, where we didn't have the profusion of specialists that places like New York or Massachusetts did, I soon found myself handling many of the pediatric endocrinology cases that came along. The focus of my lab studies now was bone growth, and I had already been closely involved with hormonal research through our work on the thymus gland. So this was a more or less natural turn of events. Endocrinologists specialize in the body's chemistry, specifically the hormonal system. That means diabetes and pituitary, adrenal, and thyroid difficulties, among other glandular diseases and syndromes. In children you are especially talking about diabetes, growth problems, and sexual disorders.

Given my nearly complete ignorance about sex when I was growing up, I still wonder sometimes exactly how it was that I became the Arkansas state expert on childhood sexual development. I think the answer is "By default." It didn't happen suddenly, but as my work progressed, referrals were coming to me, and to Ed Hughes, of course. But in 1970 Ed went off to become chief of pediatric endocrinology at the University of West Virginia, which left me. From that point on, every unusual sex case in Arkansas was showing up at my door.

In normal sexual development, both male and female embryos' sex organs begin as undifferentiated gonads. If nothing intervenes in the development of the gonads, they become ovaries. But the presence of the Y chromosome causes the gonads to become testes. The testes then produce hormones that cause the degeneration of the embryonic uterus and fallopian tubes and the development of a penis and other male structures. It's an intricate process in which one hormonal change triggers the next, which triggers the next. Along this biochemical pathway there is plenty of room for accidents and confusion. Peculiar things happen, and not as infrequently as you might suppose.

Hermaphrodites and pseudohermaphrodites aren't common, but they're not that rare either. Girls are born who look like boys, and boys who appear to be girls. Puberty can surprise you in lots of ways; the body's clock can be off by many years. Growth problems often have severe sexual consequences. By the time I got into my career development grant, I was treating all these.

True hermaphrodites sometimes have an ovary on one side and a testis on the other. Or in each of the gonads they might have an ovary and testis together—an ovatestis—while the external sexual structures might look either male or female. Pseudohermaphrodites, who appear to be one sex but are actually the other, often suffer from a condition in which hormones made by the adrenal gland are disordered, resulting in an overproduction of androgens. In baby girls the androgen causes a virilization of the external genitals. Girls with this syndrome are born with clitorises that are sometimes larger than penises and fused labia majora that look something like a scrotum. Boys with hormonal imbalances can have what is called hypospadias, a penis that is open so that it looks like a girl's labia.

I usually saw these children first as newborns. Whenever there were cases of ambiguous genitalia or any questions involving the child's sex, I got called in immediately. The first thing I'd do was order chromosome and hormonal studies, to try to determine exactly what kind of defect we were dealing with. Once I knew that, I could attempt to correct the imbalance or replace the deficient hormones. Often the treatment was successful, at which point we'd have to look at fixing up the structures surgically.

That was on relatively straightforward cases, say, when a girl baby was born with normal ovaries and a uterus but with virilized genitalia. Then it was mainly a matter of reducing the clitoral tissue and separating and shaping the labia, in addition to administering appropriate hormones. That was often the problem, since we saw far more cases of this sort in girls than in boys. But sometimes the situation wasn't anywhere near simple. Occasionally our work-ups would show a mosaic of male and female chromosomes, children who were both male and female. Then our problem was to decide which sex to make the child.

On almost all these cases I worked with John Redman, a urologist and an absolutely first-rate surgeon. John had been one of my students when I was a resident. But he wasn't the type to defer to my judgment, which was just the way I wanted it. I wasn't afraid of making decisions like this, fundamental as they were going to be to the child's life. But I was a lot more comfortable making them after thrashing them out with someone of John's caliber.

We both knew these things had to be done before the child got to be eighteen months or so. By that time, certainly by age two, the child is already beginning to think of herself or himself as a girl or boy. The child is going to be raised as one or the other, not as an it, and the identification will take some kind of psychological hold, whatever the hormones may or may not be doing.

Usually, if the child had basic external female structures, that was how we decided to go, although it seemed to me that John had a tendency to want to make boys. "Oh, I can fix this up beautifully," he'd say. "He would just make a wonderful man."

"I know you can make it pretty," I'd tell him, "but I've got to make sure it works right when this child's a teenager."

It was one thing to make a penis that looked all right. It was something else altogether to get the erectile tissue functioning, which was my point. These kids all needed ongoing hormone treatments, and I was going to be their doctor for a long time.

I had to make sure that they had working systems, and it was far easier to make a functional female than a male.

Though I followed most of these cases that we had in Arkansas from birth, on occasion John and I didn't get one until later on. Neither of us will ever forget the five-year-old who was thought to be a male and had been raised as a boy. The genitalia were more masculine than not, but when the child was eventually brought into the clinic and examined, we found ovaries, a uterus, and female chromosomes.

By that time there was no turning back. The child thought of herself as a boy, and her adrenal gland had been producing male hormone from the time of embryonic development, which had most likely had an imprinting effect on the brain. For John, this meant far more than just building complete male structures. He had to take out the vagina, uterus, and ovaries so that the boy would not end up with menstrual periods and the possibility of getting pregnant later in life.

John Redman and I might have joked with each other about who wanted to make boys and who wanted girls. But this was a serious business, and until we came to agreement on a case, we never made a move. We didn't need reminding that we were dealing with maybe *the* primary building block of self-identity. And we weren't talking about making just boys and girls, but men and women who needed to have as complete adult lives as we could give them.

Deciding on such things might have been odd in a way. Determining a person's sex doesn't feel the same as making decisions about high blood pressure or back surgery. But I don't think we ever spent too much time on the philosophical side of it. In each case a decision had to be made, and John and I happened to be the people best qualified to make it. The worst thing of all would have been not to have had clarity.

We didn't involve parents in the decision making, though we talked to them at length after we had determined what was most feasible to do. We argued it out between us; then we presented the decision to them as the best possible solution. It's very upsetting to parents when their children's genitals are abnormal.

So when you talk to them, they are really listening. More than anything they want clarity for themselves and normal, happy lives for their children.

On these deep matters of sexuality parents are looking to do everything they can for the child's benefit. I found that to be universally true in these cases of sexual extremes, as I also did counseling parents of diabetics about sex and pregnancy. That was no less so in some of the truly strange cases of precocious puberty I saw, like the two brothers whose mother brought them into the clinic one day. They were adolescent in every way, except that one was two years old and the other four.

Chapter 11

Back in Touch

I saw the two of them after the older brother had been referred to us by his preschool program. Although only four, this boy was as big as an eight-year-old. At the preschool he had been getting aggressive with the other children, pushing them down, then getting on top of them and making sexual movements. When I examined him, I found that he wasn't just big for his age; he was fully developed sexually, with axillary and pubic hair and adult-size genitals. Even more startling, his two-year-old younger brother was also well along into puberty. These two were practically babies, normal in their intellectual and emotional development and speech, a typical toddler and preschooler, except for this bizarre accident of nature that was turning them physically into men a decade before they were ready for it.

True precocious puberty is eight to ten times rarer in boys than in girls, so when you see the symptoms, you immediately suspect a tumor or some other impingement on the glandular system. But though I did a variety of studies on the two brothers, I never found anything of that nature. Nor was I able to arrest or slow their development, although we tried various medications.

I reported these cases to the NIH, and when I had exhausted our options, I made arrangements for the parents to take the boys up to Maryland for more studies and treatment. These were wonderful parents, very caring and of course extremely worried by what was happening to their boys. They were simple, poor people, though, and initially the NIH just told them to come up there with the children. I let the institutes know that these were not the kind of people who could afford to go stay in Washington, and when the officials there understood the situation, they made arrangements to take care of the whole family.

Several medical articles were written on these boys, but there wasn't any effective treatment available, and they both proceeded on through puberty. Both are adults now, short, though otherwise normal. Once they left me, they weren't my patients any longer, and I didn't have a chance to follow their development closely. But they no doubt experienced years of strangeness before the rest of the world eventually caught up with them.

Subsequently I did treat other extremely precocious children over a period of many years, and generally they did not seem especially upset by what was happening to them. There may have been some long-term effects from having been different from their peers for so long, but the actual physical changes didn't appear to bother them much. They grew fast and experienced the other normal developments of puberty, except that they were six or seven years old instead of twelve or thirteen; those younger cases, the two- and four-year-olds, were truly exceptional. Talking to these children, I always explained everything in simple terms. I told them that all of this was absolutely normal; it was just happening to them earlier than usual. Their friends might not be growing up the way they were right now, but before long they would be.

Precocious puberty usually leads to short adult stature because less growth happens before adolescence. Another problem I saw a lot of was growth hormone deficiency, which also results in short stature but often brings a host of related problems along with it. Because the pituitary secretes other trophic hormones, there is a good possibility that if someone is lacking in growth hormone, he or she may have reproductive, thyroid, and adrenal problems, in addition to difficulties in growth and maturation. People with this whole syndrome are called hypopituitary.

With all the work we were doing in the lab on the relation of growth hormone to bone metabolism, I was getting an increasingly better understanding of the complex biochemical processes that go into development. Growth problems occur statistically in about one out of every fifteen hundred people, as compared with one in five thousand for sexual abnormalities. And just as I was seeing pretty much all the sexual cases in Arkansas, I was likewise treating many of the growth problems.

These cases would ordinarily come into the University Hospital individually, but at one point I found myself treating seven boys with severe growth deficiencies at the same time. Since they were all on the ward together for several weeks, inevitably the staff began calling them the seven dwarfs although none of them was actually dwarfed in the classical sense of having disproportionate bone growth. They were just very small. They ran in age from eight to thirteen, and not one of them was more than about half his normal height.

Nowdays human growth hormone is synthesized, so there is enough to treat everybody who needs it. But when these boys were on our ward, growth hormone was a rare substance. At that time it had to be extracted from human pituitaries. Hospitals all over the country freeze-dried the pituitaries of patients whose deaths required autopsies and sent them to the National Pituitary Agency at Johns Hopkins, which purified and reconstituted the hormone. The National Pituitary Agency would allot the lyophilized hormone for studies that met its research criteria, but there wasn't enough available for therapeutic use. As a result, many growth-deficient children just couldn't be treated. They ended up as very small people lacking in various functions, even though there were certain things we could do for them with other hormones.

From that perspective, my seven patients were lucky they weren't simply growth hormone–deficient, but truly hypopituitary; they suffered from the entire syndrome of growth hormone—related problems. As a result, they fitted right into the studies I was doing, and I applied for and got quantities of the hormone from the National Pituitary Agency.

Thrown into the ward together, these children became good friends. At home, of course, they all were isolated by their diminutive size. Because what they had was so unusual, they had never seen other children like themselves, and they suffered from loneliness and feelings of low self-esteem. During the two weeks they were together, the parents got to know one another too, and many of their relationships as well as the children's friendships have lasted until now.

With these children I administered growth hormone and regulated their other hormonal imbalances. What we were doing worked, and by and large these kids grew to normal or near-normal height and made successful lives for themselves. All of them but two ended up going to college, and most married and had families. One of my "seven dwarfs" is now a successful lawyer. When I went to Washington, he liked to tell people, "You know, the surgeon general used to feel my balls." That was true, though given all the hypopituitary cases I treated, it wasn't exactly a unique distinction.

What happens is that with growth hormone patients it's important to identify the onset of puberty and assess the rate of physical maturation. With boys, the standard method of doing that is by measuring testicle volume and penis size. For this job, we use a grading system called Tanner stages. Pediatric endocrinologists all carry around with them a little instrument that has about eight or ten model testicles arranged by size as well as models representing four stages of penis growth. In each examination you judge penis development, then feel the testicles and compare them with the Tanner stage models. I'd feel; then I'd have the kids feel. "This is what I felt," I'd say. "I think it's about eight cc's. Now you feel and see if Dr. Elders got it right."

"Uh-uh, Dr. Elders," I'd hear, "I think it's more like ten."

"All right then, you feel them more often than I do. Let's say it's ten, and we'll check next visit."

By the time I started working on the NIH grant I had been out of college and on my own for almost fifteen years. In that time I hadn't exactly been a stranger in Schaal, but I didn't get down to see Mama and Daddy and the rest all that often. Months and months would sometimes pass between visits. Mama and I wrote on occasion, but that was always skimpy. And for years there was no way to talk; electrification had come in the fifties, but though it's hard to believe, I don't think the Schaal area got telephone service until the 1970s. If there was some kind of emergency, people had to use the public phone in the drugstore up in Mineral Springs.

The result was that my relationship with everyone changed from being the oldest and the everyday leader into someone who came by once in a while to say hello. My sister Pat, who was born only a couple of years before I left for college, and Phillip, who came along after, didn't know me very well, and I hardly knew them. I was their older sister, whom they'd heard about and knew of, but I wasn't really part of their lives.

Meanwhile life wasn't standing still for my sisters and brothers any more than it was for me. As they grew up, all the kids started scattering, which was probably inevitable given how hard things were in Schaal. After high school Katie moved to Detroit, where she got a good job at Ford and started getting promoted up the ladder. Beryl eventually followed her there and also got a job at Ford. Charles went to work for GM in Chicago, where several of Daddy's brothers and sisters had established themselves earlier. Bernard and Chester left too, to embark on their own lives—Bernard even before he finished high school.

But even though we were scattered and not in touch all that much, my feelings about most of my brothers and sisters were set in stone by everything we had been through together. For years Katie and I had changed their diapers and carted them around and looked after them. I had worked out in our fields with everyone except Pat and Phillip. And when I did visit home, I couldn't help feeling like a mother even toward Phillip, which I'm sure annoyed him considerably since he already had one mother to tell him what to do.

If anything, my protective feelings got even stronger over the years. I think part of that came from seeing them in situations that I had left behind and that now seemed to me so hard and pitiful, even if they hadn't struck me that way when I was younger and living through them myself. Some things I wished I had never seen—like Mama and some of them hiring themselves out as migrant farm workers. That was something I never had to do myself, other than picking peaches, which was a nice easy job in the vicinity of home.

They really started going out as migrants after I left. Mama, Charles, Bernard, and usually Chester, who was only a boy but could pick cotton and anything else you put him on better than most men, would go out on the trucks to farms in Arizona and California, traveling a thousand miles day and night, packed with the rest of a work crew into somebody's flatbed stake truck half covered over by a canvas for shade. The trucks ran twenty-four hours with two drivers switching off. They'd make stops at gas stations to use bathrooms and buy snacks, but other than that they just kept rolling. When they got to the work, they'd stay a month or more sometimes, living in camps and sleeping on sacks they filled with picked cotton.

Once I visited them in Ohio, where they were working the tomato harvest. I was in medical school then, and I had a summer job as a physical therapist at a camp for handicapped children in western Massachusetts. I must have had a few days off or something, so I traveled out to where they were working. That particular day it was raining buckets, and the roads were swamped. When I finally got to the place, there were all these farm workers living in pup tents in the middle of a sea of mud. Some people were trying to cook over smoldering wood that was about the best you could do toward a campfire that day, but mostly they just seemed to be walking around in the mud and water. The place had no privies or any other facilities. There was a hydrant down the road they could get drinking water from, but that was it. The rest was just mud and people wandering aimlessly.

I tried not to act sad when I found Mama and Chester and Uncle Buh, who was also there. But I was very down. All I could think was that I had to try to get them out, so they would never have to do this to survive. I did not want my sisters and brothers growing up living this way. That thought was very forceful to me, very vivid. I watched the men sitting around, my uncle and his friends, the water raining down on them, mud everywhere. I remember that I wasn't thinking so much right then about Buh or even Mama. I was thinking about Chester and Bernard and the others and how to keep this from happening to them anymore.

Of course I wasn't actually able to do anything then, but later, when I was earning a salary, that changed, especially when some of them began thinking about college. Oliver felt exactly like I did. If somebody wanted to go to school, we would somehow get the money for it, whether we had to go borrow it or what. We wouldn't give money to buy a car, but we would always have money for tuition.

Starting in about 1965, just after Kevin was born, my sister Pat began attending the University of Arkansas up in Fayetteville. Summers she stayed with us while she worked at the University Hospital, where I got her a job. Then after a couple of years she transferred to the nursing school in Little Rock, so she was with us most of the time.

Having Pat around gave me a chance to remeet her. Except for my once-in-a-while visits, the last real time I had spent with Pat was when she was three years old. Pat had lived a lot of her childhood and teenage years with Aunt Jo and Uncle Tommy up in Kansas City, to the extent that she was really like a daughter to them. One result was that I didn't see her much even when I did go home. Now that she was almost adult, she had turned out vivacious and quick-witted. She was also strikingly beautiful, so much so that one year she was elected queen of the school of medicine.

Pat had a penchant for digging up old stories about the family and what it was like in the old days. That may have partly been because she had not spent all that much time on the farm herself, but I also think she just had a natural fascination with such things. I can't say that I shared her curiosity at the time, though now, of course, I wish I had. I felt like I had lived through those old days personally, and there wasn't much about them that I wanted to reacquaint myself with. I was glad to be rid of them.

Pat finished her preclinical work at the nursing school, but despite how bright she was, she struggled through the last part of her studies. Finally it was pretty clear that she wasn't going to make it, and six weeks before the end of her senior semester, the school dropped her out. We all had a hard time with that, maybe me especially. But in retrospect it seemed to me that she just couldn't have been all that interested in nursing. She may not have known at that point what she wanted to do, but her years in school had convinced her that nursing wasn't a profession she was called to.

Not long after this Pat decided to go up to Michigan, where she could stay with Katie. While she was there she finished her bachelor's degree at the University of Detroit, then started working toward a doctorate in linguistics and folklore at the University of Michigan. That was a total switch from what she had done before. But it built on her natural bent, as everybody in the family knew whom she had ever gotten after with all her questions. "Do you remember such and such?" she'd ask Chester, who had left the farm the minute he had enough money to get himself to Kansas. "Was that the way it really was?"

"Well," he'd say, "who cares if it was? I'm trying to get away from all that."

"What about old so-and-so?" she'd ask me or Reva or Buh, only to hear, "Pat, what in the world do you want to sit around and talk about dead folks for?"

But Pat was insatiable, so it didn't completely surprise anyone that she went on to graduate school. For her dissertation she started what became a continuing study of the Gullah culture on South Carolina's offshore islands, where native African traditions endured much more persistently than they did among other African Americans. She interviewed old-time storytellers, collected their tales, and recorded their speech patterns. Then she started visiting Africa and identifying the roots of the language and customs she was noting among the island people.

Pat worked hard on that doctorate and was very proud of what she had accomplished, which she had good reason to be. She had found her vocation. Her work was beautifully done and eventually gained wide recognition. Once, later on, when she was a professor at Howard University and I was visiting Washington, I introduced her at some gathering as "my sister Pat Jackson." Afterward she said, "Dear sister, I'm Dr. Jackson, and I would appreciate it if when you introduce me to people you would tell them that."

I said, "Yes, ma'am. I'll make sure I remember that."

And I did too.

———

In 1972, a couple of years after Pat had left, Oliver and I decided to move. Eric was nine and Kevin seven, and the house seemed to be shrinking around us. We needed something bigger. Besides, we had been transporting them up to elementary school in Lakewood, which was a community a couple of miles away that had better schools. Also, for the first time in our lives we had enough income to afford something we'd really like. So we started house hunting.

Our search for a new house wasn't exactly a shining chapter in my personal history of race relations. We were working with a white realtor named Eloise Odum who dealt mainly in upper-level houses in North Little Rock. Eloise was an excellent, professional person who was committed to getting us something we wanted. Among the houses we saw was one we really liked in a brand-new upscale neighborhood. But when we started talking to the builder about it, he put us off to the investment company that was financing the construction, and we eventually heard that they would rather not sell it to us. No reason was given, but everyone involved understood perfectly well what was going on.

That upset Eloise considerably, and she got really determined.

Then we looked at a house out in West Little Rock that we wanted to buy. But in the end the owners wouldn't sell us that one either. Finally Eloise had a listing in Lakewood, the neighborhood where the boys were going to school. This house was just sitting there empty; the owners had moved out already.

Oliver and I weren't wild about it. But it was big enough and well built, and it was on a little peninsula that jutted out into a lake, so the surroundings were beautiful. The house was listed at seventy thousand, but when word got around that a black family was thinking about moving into the neighborhood, prices started dropping like a shot bird. Maybe people were imagining some kind of mass migration, I don't know. But in the end we got it for forty-seven thousand. The owners were so eager to sell that they agreed to pay the closing costs.

That wasn't the end of it, though. After we had signed the purchase and sale agreement, we couldn't find anybody who would give us a mortgage. I was an associate professor by then, and Oliver was a teacher with seniority, so we both were doing well. We were a two-income professional family, but somehow the mortgage market just seemed to have dried right up. Finally, after a couple of months of looking, Eloise's real estate company decided to finance it themselves. So we got the house. But it wasn't a great experience, and to top it off, we began to hear that the neighbors were pretty nipped that we were moving in there, though of course they didn't know us any better than we knew them. I can't imagine what they might have thought when we finally did show up; Oliver's basketball team moved us, which might really have looked like an invasion.

Relations weren't exactly cold at first, just kind of distant. At one point we were having some furniture delivered during the working day, and I asked the lady next door, Mrs. Seemel, if she could let the delivery people in. Well, it turned out she was going to be busy with something else, so she couldn't do it. That was fine, of course, but it more or less reflected the general temperature.

Then about a month after that Oliver and I were having a big party for his fraternity. I had been held up at the hospital all day, and by the time I got home I knew we didn't have time to get everything done without help. When I looked outside, Mr. and Mrs. Seemel were straightening up their yard. They looked like just what I needed at that moment, so I marched out and said, "Mrs. Seemel, I need you and Mr. Seemel to come help me." I think they were shocked. They stared at me, and their mouths were working, but they didn't quite know how to say no.

"Well, what do you want me to do?" Mrs. Seemel asked.

"Your yard looks fine," I said. "I need you to come inside."

So she came in and started fixing salad while I had Mr. Seemel running around putting out tables. I just kind of shanghaied them.

Then I said, "Listen, since you're here already, why don't you just stay for the party?"

And they said, "Oh, well, no . . . we couldn't . . . I mean, we don't look . . . we aren't dressed. . . ."

So I said, "Well, I think you look just fine. Please sit down and stay awhile."

By that time Oliver's fraternity brothers were already arriving, and the Seemels stayed, and soon they were just part of the party. They had a real good time, which broke the ice permanently. After that they became some of our best friends on the block.

But not our only friends. There was a retired Army colonel and his wife who lived next door on the other side who did the same thing to us that I had done to the Seemels. They were putting on a big wedding in their backyard for one of their children, and they needed some emergency help, so they grabbed Oliver and me. We had to run over and spend the afternoon helping them take care of their wedding. I thought, This is getting to be like some kind of neighborhood ritual. Then there was a pediatrician I'd known for a long time who lived down the block. Another doctor lived down that way too, a surgeon who had young children around Eric and Kevin's age. The surgeon's children always seemed to be up at our house, and ours were always at their house. So that worked out. The man whose parents had actually built our house lived across the street, and a pediatric dentist lived directly opposite us. Later his son studied medicine, and he made rounds with me on the pediatric ward just this past summer. So we soon got to know all our neighbors, and they all seemed really very nice and friendly, even though they'd been unhappy about our moving to that street at first and our presence might have taken them a little getting used to.

———

Not long after we moved to Lakewood my brother Bernard came to town. Bernard had left the farm early, when he was fourteen or fifteen. The story that got back to us later was that my father had gotten into a shouting argument with somebody that happened to take place in the field opposite Bernard's girl-friend's house. Bernard was so mortified that he stopped doing whatever he was doing and went back home. When everybody else came in for supper, Bernard wasn't there. He had just disap-peared. Awhile later they heard he was up with Aunt Jo in Kansas City.

From Kansas City Bernard went to stay with Katie in Detroit. A little while later he got a job as house boy to the Englanders, a wealthy Jewish furniture-manufacturing family. When the Englanders learned he didn't have his diploma, they became very insistent about his going back to school. After Bernard moved to Little Rock, he told me the story and laughed. "I said I didn't want to go back yet, and they said that in that case I'd have to find another job. They just wouldn't let you stay around there unless you went to school. They'd fire you."

So Bernard worked for the Englanders and studied for his GED. Once he had that he signed up for the Army and trained as a paratrooper. By then he was also thinking about college. Eventually, between the GI Bill and what we were able to help with, he had enough money so that he finished his enlistment and enrolled at Tennessee A&I. Of course Bernard was used to animals from the farm, the same as the rest of us. He had always worked real well with them and loved them. So it wasn't sur-prising that when he finished college, he applied to the Tuskegee

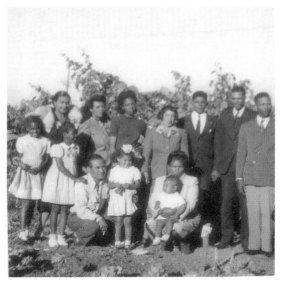

Mother, with baby Chester, and Dad *(third from right)* in California, 1940s

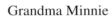Grandma Minnie

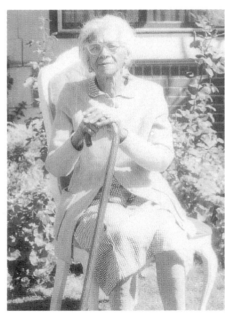

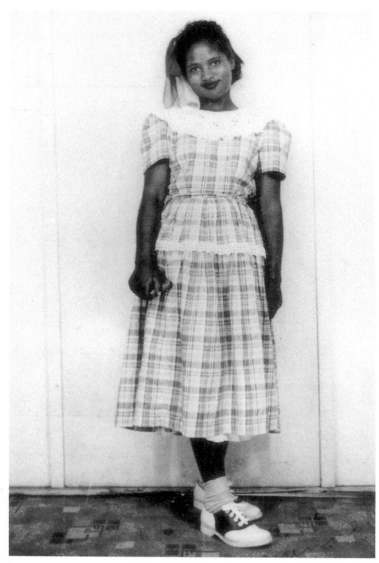

Age fifteen, ready for college

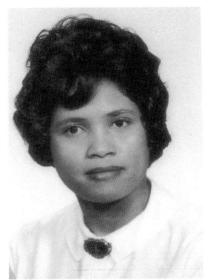

College student

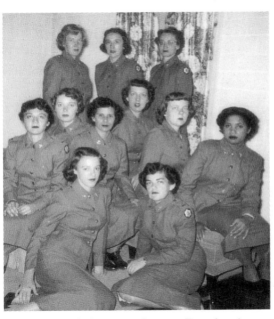

My physical therapy class at Brooke Army
Center, 1953

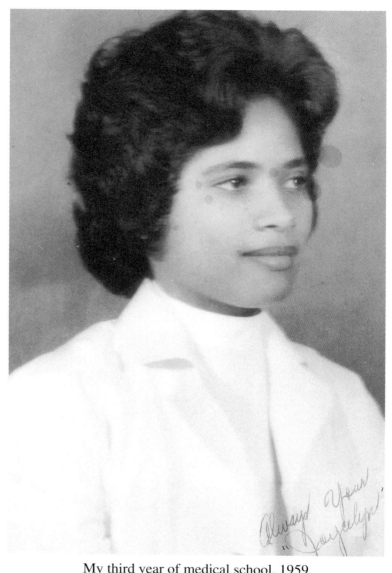

My third year of medical school, 1959

Medical school graduate, with Dr. Brown *(left)* and my father, 1960

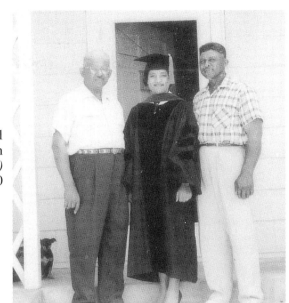

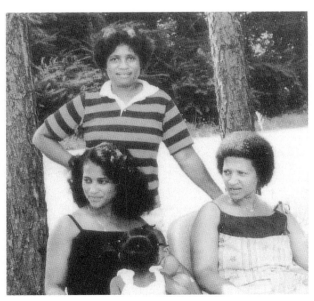

With my sisters Pat *(left)* and Beryl

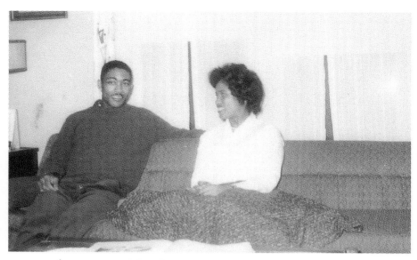

With Oliver in our first home

A formal occasion at the
University of Minnesota,
where I was a pediatric
intern

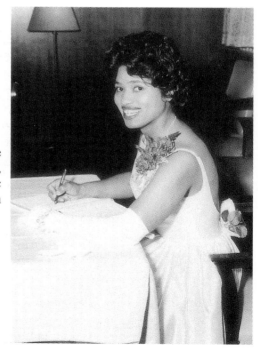

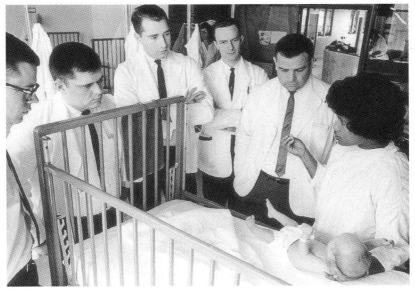

On teaching rounds at the University of Arkansas Medical School when I was chief resident

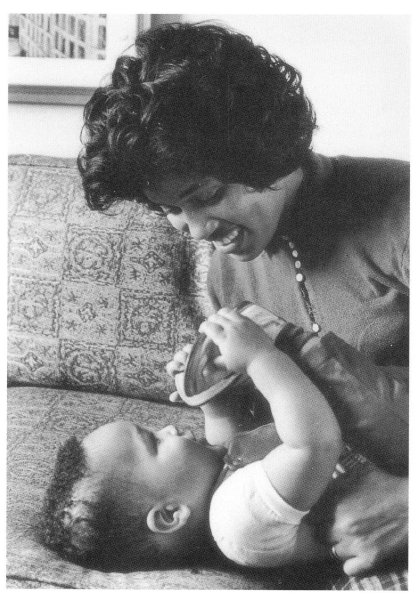

Private time with my son Eric, 1963

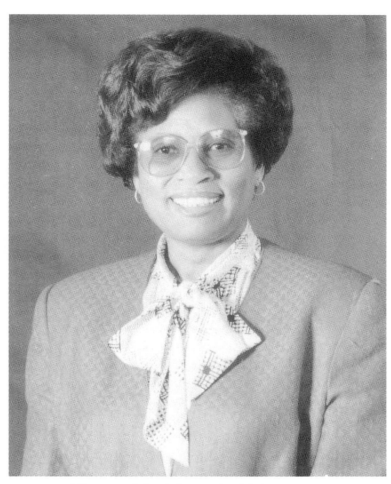

Director of the Arkansas health department

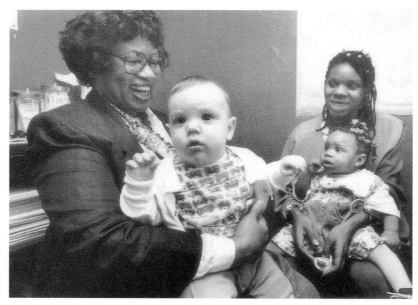

With my patients at the clinic in Little Rock's Central High School

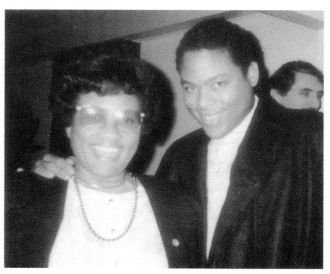

Kevin graduating from Grambling with an M.B.A.

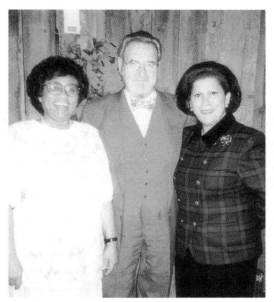

Two former surgeons general and one nominee: C. Everett Koop stands between me and Toni Novello.

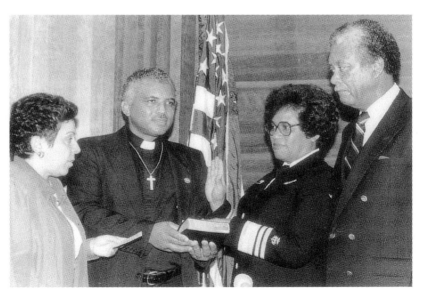

Chester swears me in as surgeon general. Donna Shalala on the left, Oliver on the right.

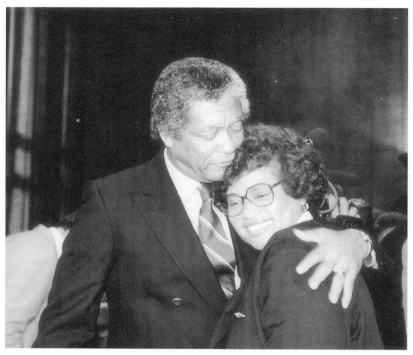

With Oliver after my confirmation as surgeon general

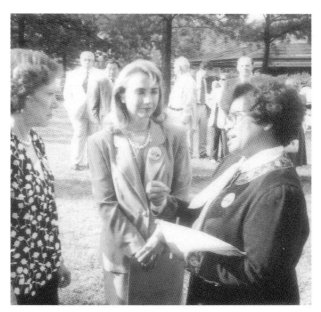

With Rosalynn Carter and Hillary Clinton

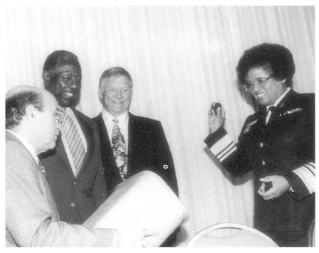

Photo opportunity with Joe Garagiola, Hank Aaron,
and Mickey Mantle in 1994

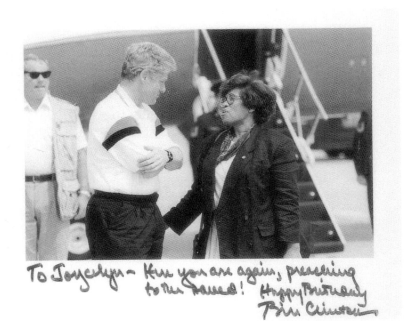

With Bill Clinton. "Here you are again, preaching to the saved!"

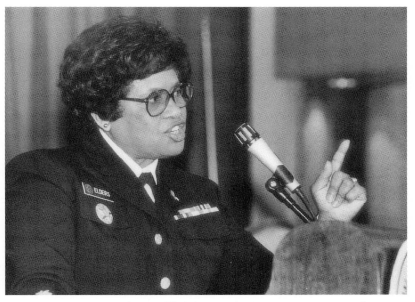

During one of my official speeches as surgeon general

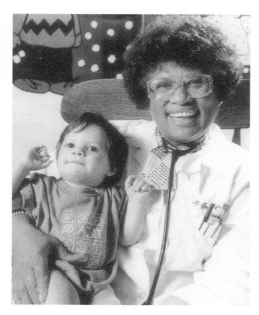

In the clinic with a young patient after leaving Washington

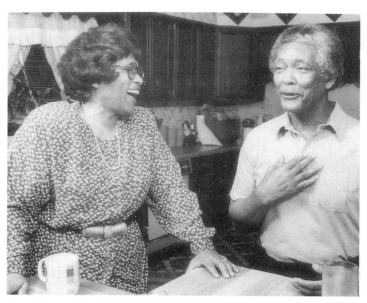

Back home in Little Rock with Oliver after my resignation

University veterinary school. When he completed that, he went on to specialize in animal dermatology and joined the faculty at Tuskegee, not bad for someone who had dropped out of high school at fourteen.

Bernard taught veterinary medicine for several years, but he was looking to go into practice, and I was encouraging him to come back to Arkansas. In 1973, he did. He bought a going practice from a Little Rock vet who was retiring, and before long business was booming.

Bernard was the first and only black veterinarian in Arkansas. There were plenty of black farmers in Arkansas, but extremely few of them even had money for doctors, let alone veterinarians. If their big animals got that sick, they mainly shot them. And Arkansas's urban black community wasn't nearly as large as that in some nearby states, which meant that it would have been harder for a black vet to sustain a practice in Little Rock than someplace like Memphis or Dallas. But between the previous doctor's clientele and Bernard's reputation in the black community, his practice was as mixed as you could get. He drew from all over.

It didn't take Bernard that long to become one of the more visible black professionals in Little Rock. He had a successful practice, he got along well with everyone, and he was unusually handsome (Chester says that Bernard and Pat inherited all the good-looking genes in the family). He also had a flamboyant way about him. With no wife and no children and not even his own house for several years, he was a well-to-do bachelor with no obligations. So Bernard spent his money on sports cars and boats and other visible acquisitions. He lived large. *Ebony* wrote an article on him as one of the most prominent and eligible black bachelors in the country.

When Bernard did finally buy a house, it was only five or six blocks from ours. He stopped by every morning for breakfast and often came to have dinner with us. He'd drive up in one of his new cars, and Eric and Kevin would just stare. They were sure that he was a millionaire, because by contrast we were obviously poor as church mice.

To the boys Bernard was a kind of phenomenon. He not only had the latest things, but was generous and warm and funny—the kind of person they could show off to their friends, all of whom quickly took to calling him Uncle Bernard too. Somehow the name stuck, and after a while it seemed like everybody in Little Rock was calling him Uncle Bernard. Sunday afternoons Bernard took the boys out on his boat, and often as not half the kids in the neighborhood would go along with them. Weekday mornings he liked to come by just after dawn to pick Eric up; one was as crazy about fishing as the other.

In 1976 Bernard met and married Bernita Terry, who was a lawyer and worked as an attorney for the city of Little Rock. Bernita may not have been the first black woman to have held such a significant position in the city government, but if not, she was close to it. With professions they enjoyed and plenty of income, it would have been hard to find anyone with better prospects for happiness and a good life.

But there was one disturbing element that I began to hear about after a while, something about a former acquaintance of Bernita's from law school who was bothering her and Bernard. I didn't know how to judge the things that Bernard was telling me when he dropped by for breakfast. I couldn't even tell how seriously he and Bernita took it at first. But a kind of cloud of threat began to hang over them.

Chapter 12

Losses

❦

What I began picking up from Bernard was that this person from Bernita's past was obsessed with her. It was somebody she had known in law school, not an old boyfriend, he said, just an acquaintance. Now this individual lived in Little Rock. He had begun calling and writing letters, threatening Bernard.

I didn't know what to think. Bernard didn't talk about it much; he just let little bits and pieces of information drop now and then. Even then he seemed more annoyed than upset. To me the whole thing had a vague quality to it. I wasn't sure how long this had been going on or even what it was exactly that was going on. Had this person been obsessed with Bernita for years? Had he followed her around since law school, or was this some kind of recent development? Was he stalking her? I knew Bernard wouldn't have been making something like this up, but I couldn't get a grasp on how seriously he was taking the whole thing. He wasn't a person to get upset about too much, and whenever he mentioned something or other, he seemed almost embarrassed that he was paying it any attention. It was clear something uncomfortable was going on, but I didn't get the sense of any kind of great, imminent danger.

But as time passed, I began to hear more. Bernard let slip one day that some of the letters he was getting included death threats. One envelope had a bullet with his name engraved on it. Then strange things started happening around Bernard's house. Sometimes he and Bernita would come home from an evening out and find that someone had been inside. Nothing was ever taken, but things would be moved around, as if someone had wanted to let them know how vulnerable they were.

Finally Bernita got so frightened that they went out and got a restraining order. Bernard still wasn't eager to make a big thing out of it by pressing charges. He probably thought the restraining order would be enough to keep this person away. Besides, with Bernita being a city attorney they were well connected downtown, which gave them an extra little sense of security. Then, not long after the order had been issued, Bernard's boat mysteriously blew up. The boat was up on blocks in his front yard when one night an explosion rocked the whole neighborhood and left the boat a wrecked, blackened mess.

One evening in April I was out canvassing the neighborhood for a cystic fibrosis drive. I was chairman of the drive that year, and for several hours I was running all around Lakewood, stopping by people's homes to check on the volunteers and collect contributions. When I got home, I was exhausted. Oliver wasn't back from practice yet, so instead of fixing dinner, I just kicked off my shoes and made myself a cup of coffee. While I was sitting there in the lounger reading the paper I hadn't had time to look at that morning, the phone rang. When I picked it up, Bernita's mother was on the other end. Her voice was shaking. Something terrible had happened, she said. I should come over immediately. No one knew if Bernard was all right or not.

I raced over to Bernard's house with the blood pounding in my ears. When I got there, the door was opened, and it seemed like most of Bernita's family was inside: her mother, her sisters and brother. Half of them were trying to calm her down, but without much success. She was wildly agitated, almost in a state of hysteria. She had come home from an evening art class sometime earlier and found Bernard tied up on the floor. While she was standing there staring, her stalker had jumped out at her from the next room and put a gun to her head. Then he tied her up, untied Bernard except for his hands, and forced Bernard out of the house with him. The two of them had driven off in Bernard's Jeep. As soon as Bernita got herself loose, she called the police. They had been there taking her statement a little before I arrived. An all-points bulletin was out for the man and Bernard and for the Jeep.

While Bernita's mother was telling me this, I began to remember that sometime that night while I was driving around canvassing I had seen Bernard's Jeep. Bernard had a fancy top-of-the-line white and gray model that was hard to miss. Somewhere or other I had seen that Jeep parked, or one that looked exactly like it. I hadn't stopped to look, but somehow the picture of it had stayed in my head. I couldn't recall where, maybe somewhere near the mall, I thought, but I had definitely seen it.

Right then Oliver walked in the door. I have no idea how he knew to come there. After Bernita's mother's call I don't think I had the presence of mind to leave a note. But there he was, along with a neighbor of ours. While I was hustling them out to the car, I explained to them what had happened. Whether I was completely coherent or not I don't know, but they got the idea pretty quickly that we had to find Bernard's Jeep as fast as we could.

With Oliver driving I did my best to retrace the routes I had taken through Lakewood earlier that evening. But I had been out for hours, crisscrossing the whole area, and I couldn't really remember all the streets I had been on or in what order I had driven them. We cruised for more than an hour. We must have been down every road in Lakewood, but we didn't have any luck. Hard as I racked my brain, I just could not recall where it was I had seen that Jeep. Finally there was nothing to do but go home and wait.

That night there was no sleeping. I called my brothers and sisters to let them know what was going on. I also called my parents, as badly as I hated to do that before we had any definite information. But by now Bernard's abduction was all over the local news, and I didn't want them picking it up from radio or television. Once that was done, Oliver and I just sat there and choked on the tension. I could feel them all out there waiting next to their telephones: Katie and Pat and Beryl and Charles in Michigan; Chester in Louisville, Kentucky, where he was a pastor; Mama and Daddy and Phillip down home in Schaal. I was getting so tight and hot I thought something might just burst.

It wasn't until the next morning that we got a call. Bernard's Jeep had been located, with Bernard sitting in the passenger-side seat, dead. A family that lived out by the mall had noticed the Jeep parked in front of their house the night before. They hadn't thought anything about it, but the next morning the Jeep was still there. One of the family's sons went to check it out; he was interested in having a close-up look at an unusual car like that. When he looked inside, there was Bernard slumped over in the seat, shot once behind the ear.

Later that morning the police picked up the killer. They knew who it was, and they didn't have much trouble tracking him down. But that wasn't the slightest relief to anyone at all. I especially didn't know what we were going to do about Mama. Daddy was being his usual stoic self, though God knows what must have been going on inside. But Mama was inconsolable. When everyone started arriving for the funeral, our grief over Bernard was distracted by worry about Mama. All she seemed able to say was "Now that Bern's gone, I might as well die too."

I finally told her, "Mama, you're spending all your time worrying about the one who's lost. But you've got seven more. God left you here for some reason, and it was so you could take care of the rest of us. So that's what you've got to start doing."

The funeral was held at Bernita's church, even though Bernard had converted to Catholicism sometime before he arrived in Little Rock and often went to services at St. Patrick's on weekdays as well as Sundays. But many people from his congregation were there, as well as Bernard's fraternity brothers and a large mix of people from both the black and white communities. In everything he did Bernard had won people to him. You could truthfully say about him that he had only friends and not an enemy in the world, except for the man who killed him. There was something unbelievable about losing Bernard. It was so awful to think that someone could live such a completely kind and friendly life yet be struck down the way he was.

Bill Clinton was also at the funeral. At that time Clinton was a smart young political star in his first term as governor. I had met him earlier, when he was still attorney general, at a political gathering held by my friends the Stancils, who lived a street over from us in Lakewood. Clinton had been there with Hillary, so I met her too, though it was a big party with lots of people milling around and lots of politicians, and I can't say that either they or I made much of an impression on each other.

But when Bernard died, Clinton was already governor. A short time before this he had asked me to serve on the Arkansas Industrial Development Commission, though I still didn't know him other than to say hello. I thought it was very considerate of him to come to the funeral. Not that there was anything unusual about Clinton's visiting black churches and going to black funerals. Arkansas's black community was part of his constituency, and that was something he did often. Chester says that Bill Clinton has probably attended ten times more funerals than any other President in history. However that may be, for him to come to the funeral for Bernard meant something to all of us.

Bernard's killer faced a charge of first-degree murder, which in Arkansas at that time meant either a death sentence or life without parole. The prosecutor's office was pressing for the death penalty, and Bernita wanted that too. But when I was asked about it, I testified that Bernard would have been absolutely against putting this man to death. I told the judge that if the man needed blood, Bernard would have lain down and given it to him.

In fact I think every one of my sisters and brothers would be opposed to capital punishment on principle. I was deeply opposed to it, even though this wasn't a subject I had ever had many discussions about. In court I didn't discuss my own views, only what I felt Bernard's position would have been. But I had always been upset by the idea of judicial killing. Our own terrible situation, with this deranged person on trial for Bernard's death, didn't do anything to change my opinion. I knew most of the arguments, pro and con, but nothing I had heard or read had ever changed my natural inclination on this. I just did not believe, either before then or now that this had happened to Bernard, that any of us is good enough to make the decision to kill somebody else. On this subject my instincts said that you should not be able to take away something you can't give and that putting someone to death for having put someone else to death isn't something an intelligent society will do. You want your community to embody principles of decency and humaneness, and to kill for revenge or punishment has always struck me as something out of our lower instincts. Even animals don't do such things, and when we do them, we diminish ourselves dreadfully. I thought that then and I still think it, even if I didn't say it in court.

The jury convicted Bernard's killer and sentenced him to life without parole. He has been in prison since, the last I heard in some kind of behavioral unit in Pine Bluff. I know that because a number of years ago he somehow found out that Chester was the Methodist superintendent in that area and wrote a letter to him. It wasn't something Chester wanted to get, any more than the rest of us wanted to hear about it. The pain this man caused still lies heavy on us all, even though it's been almost ten years now. None of us wanted him put to death, but I can't say there's much forgiveness in our hearts either.

———

Bernard's was the first death Eric and Kevin experienced close up. To me it seemed that they grieved for him, then began to recover, though trying to deal with my own pain probably didn't make me that wonderful an observer.

Eric was fifteen at the time, a sophomore at Northeast High School, and Kevin was thirteen, almost ready to leave junior high. Both of them were such good children that I used to run around and brag about how easy it was to raise boys, how it was just wonderful and no problem. Others might be complaining that their sons were rambunctious and troublesome, but Oliver and I never had any of that. We'd hear about sibling rivalry and how someone else's boys were always fighting and getting at each other. But that didn't happen in our house. Eric had really liked Kevin from the time he was a baby, and Kevin adored Eric, which was probably more natural. What we mainly had with the boys was harmony. Later on in life my opinions about raising boys changed. I began to think God knew that back then I didn't understand how to cope and I wouldn't have been able to handle it. So He waited until I could handle it, then gave it to me all at once.

In December 1993 the story of Kevin's drug problems surfaced when he was arrested for selling an eighth of an ounce of cocaine to a police informant. Because I was surgeon general then, the situation made all the front pages. Two and a half years later we still haven't seen the end of a long legal fight over how Kevin became a target and whether the police entrapped him. A lot of strange things went into Kevin's arrest that have made people suspicious of exactly what happened. Through this whole thing I have tried to resist the idea that Kevin may have been a victim of my association with the President. But given the rage and pure vindictiveness some Arkansas Republicans feel toward Bill Clinton, it's hard to keep from making connections.

None of which is to say that Kevin's problems weren't real. They were, and they put Oliver and me through emotions we never expected to have. It's a harsh experience watching your child struggle with addiction, then go through incarceration. At times we have felt frustrated and desperate. We've also been hopeful, and I can even say thankful. During our own troubles the actor Carroll O'Connor's son committed suicide because of his addiction. Addicts die of overdoses every day. I have no doubt whatsoever that if Kevin's problems hadn't come to light, we might have lost him. As it's turned out so far, we only lost him to prison for a while. And as hard as that was for Oliver and me to accept, even prison had its positive side.

Recovering addicts say that once you've been addicted, you are always an addict, no matter how long you might have stayed sober. They say you have no alternative but to take one day at a time. I'm not an expert on addiction, but I don't feel I have a lot of illusions about it either. I know that Kevin is going to need a lifetime's worth of determination to see himself through. But I have hopes that he will make it. I've always felt that with all his difficulties, Kevin is a super human being. I like the inner stuff that both my children have. I know that inside, they're good people.

That's true of both of them, but I always tell people that Kevin is absolutely the best one of us all. Eric is more like Oliver and me in that we're strong-willed people who like to do things our own way. In our family it was always Kevin who reached out to help the others. I could see that from very early on, when Eric would want the biggest and the best of whatever there was, and instead of objecting, Kevin would be trying to find a way to give it to him. Kevin was always unselfish, always giving and doing his best to be good.

By the time we moved to Lakewood, Oliver and I had bought up several rental houses, which we'd often get for a low price because they needed fixing up. Before long this became a kind of sideline for the family. In our spare time we all worked on these properties. But when we did, Oliver and Eric and I each had a tendency to go off and do our own thing, whether it was cleaning or painting or putting up wallboard or whatever. There was always enough to do in these places so that you could carve out your own territory and stick to it, which was one of the reasons we liked the work. If I'd go to help someone, it would be for a minute; then I'd want to be back doing what I wanted to do. Eric, Oliver, and I liked to be the leaders. But Kevin was always there to lend a hand to us and do the things the rest of us didn't want to.

By the time he was fourteen and fifteen Kevin was handling all the money from these properties. He collected the rent and made the bank deposits and ran around taking care of everything that needed it. Oliver and I really thought that if something happened to us, Kevin would just take over and run the properties. He was like a mother hen. He felt responsible, and he never hesitated putting other people's needs in front of his own.

Maybe the reason I didn't see this as a sign of trouble was that in that respect I thought Kevin had a lot of me in him. If someone had asked me to characterize my own childhood, I would have said that two of the main things were taking responsibility and pleasing everybody else before I thought about pleasing myself. But whether it was from me or somewhere else, Kevin clearly had a need to take care of people. Eric most likely would never have gotten into college if Kevin hadn't filled out his application for him. When he did get in, Kevin packed him up, drove him there, and got him set up. "When I'm ready to go away to college," he told me, "I guess I'm just gonna have to put you and Daddy into a nursing home."

Now, looking back on it, I think that maybe part of Kevin's compulsiveness about helping stemmed from loneliness. In Glenview, the black neighborhood we had come from, every house had three or four kids. Children were everywhere, all the time. On Halloween we'd have sixty trick-or-treaters at our door. In Lakewood every child we knew came to the door too, but it was never more than eight or ten. Lakewood might have been the best neighborhood in North Little Rock, but it was mainly a community of affluent, older people. There just weren't that many children around.

When Kevin was five and six, I tried to compensate by being with him as much as I could. I had taken a part-time position as supervisory doctor at a large nursing and convalescent home, and when I'd make visits there, I'd put a little white jacket on him and bring him along. On weekends he'd come to the hospital with me and join the squad of residents and interns that trailed after me making rounds. We did everything we could to put Kevin, and Eric too, together with kids their age, to give them activities they liked and help them along with what they wanted to do. Kevin took piano lessons three times a week from a woman in the neighborhood. Fall was youth football time, and in the spring there was baseball. There were Cub Scouts and after that Boy Scouts. But when he wasn't busy, the only thing Kevin seemed to do was sit in front of the TV and eat. He didn't eat that much at meals, but he ate all night.

Years later I wondered whether it would have made a difference to Kevin if we had stayed in a black neighborhood. That was something Oliver and I might not have been too conscious of at the time. Neither of us had ever felt separated in the least from the black community, regardless of what color Lakewood was. No one was ever going to take Schaal out of me, no more than anyone was going to take De Witt out of Oliver. By this time Oliver was teaching and coaching in integrated Hall High School rather than segregated Horace Mann, and my work setting was mostly white. But that had hardly split us off from our roots or our black church or our black friends. It wasn't something we even particularly thought about.

But there was no question that our children were growing up differently. Eric had gone to Montessori, where there might have been two or three other black children. Then his elementary school and high school had been mainly white. Now he lived in Lakewood, where most of his friends were white. From what we could see, Eric was never uncomfortable with any of that. He just adapted. He played football and started weight lifting and bodybuilding when he was thirteen or so, which became a lifelong avocation. He had an easy way about him and lots of friends. He seemed at home with everyone.

Kevin was different. I don't know if it was because he had been in a black day-care center at Horace Mann or that he had spent a year in the mostly black elementary school in Glenview. But it sometimes seemed like in Lakewood he was missing something. He had a couple of black teachers in the Lakewood elementary school who had made him feel really special. Even after he was no longer at that school, Kevin would get on his bicycle in the afternoon and go up there to see about those teachers. But that was probably because he didn't have any real friends to come home and play with in the neighborhood. At school he hung out a lot with the black kids who had been bused in. But after hours he didn't have a way to get down to their neighborhood, and they didn't have a way to get to his. So even if they wanted to stop off and visit, it wasn't really possible.

I don't think the fact that he was a black boy in a mostly white world was what made Kevin lonely. But standing out like that could well have made him feel even more self-conscious and separate than he already did. In mulling over these things later in life, I've often thought that he'd maybe have been happier or better off if we had stayed in the old neighborhood. Maybe he would have had more friendships. Maybe they would have been stronger.

Something that added to Kevin's difficulties from the time he was young, and was also the most obvious sign of them, was his weight. What initiated that, I think, was the bout he had with acute glomerulonephritis when he was four. Although many people may not have heard of it, glomerulonephritis, which is also called Bright's disease, isn't that uncommon. It's brought on by a streptococcal infection that affects the kidneys and causes severe inflammation, swelling, and high blood pressure. Most often the infection clears up completely and you never have any more trouble with it. But about 10 percent of the cases suffer complications, which can be severe. Renal failure, seizures, hypertensive encephalopathy, and even heart failure are all possibilities.

It can be a frightening business. Knowing what I knew, I kept Kevin quiet. I didn't let him run around and play. I didn't want him to exercise or do anything that might stress his system. He was very good about that. He didn't do anything except sit around and eat.

Long after the nephritis was gone the eating continued. Kevin got to be very heavy, so much so that from the time he was seven or eight we took him up to West Stockbridge, Massachusetts, every summer to a fat camp. He always lost forty or fifty pounds there, but then by Christmas he'd have gained it all back. By the time he was sixteen he weighed over three hundred pounds.

It affected him. Kevin had a car and enough money, and he always seemed to feel like he had to go drive people around and buy the potato chips and Coke and cookies. To me it looked like he was reaching out to people every way he could, trying to attract friends with favors and generosity. I never felt that many friends reaching for Kevin.

At the same time I may have been too protective in how much I wanted to give Eric and Kevin, though that wasn't obvious to me at the time. What I knew for sure was that I never wanted my children to go through what I had gone through. I didn't want them to have to work like I did or to worry about how to scrape up a nickel or about how they were going to go to school. I remembered the agony of not knowing how to pay my room and board or where I was going to get the money for a notebook and pencil. I never wanted my children ever to have to think about anything like that. I considered all those material things to be my job and Oliver's. Eric and Kevin grew up knowing that all they had to do was hint they might need something and the chances were pretty good they were going to get it.

I also knew that when the time came, there was a way to deal with Kevin's obesity. When it was clear he wasn't going to be able to lose the weight himself, I decided that when he finished high school, I would have his stomach stapled. I had friends at the hospital who could do that, along with whatever tissue reductions were necessary. The stomach operation reduces the size of the stomach so that the person can ingest only a small amount of food at a time. If he tries to swallow more than half a cup at a meal, it comes back up. Stomach stapling is a last-ditch approach to obesity, but it often works. It did with Kevin. After the stapling was done, he lost almost two hundred pounds.

But while the operation worked, neither Oliver nor I really addressed the underlying problem. We weren't asking ourselves why it was that Kevin needed to do what he was doing, so that maybe we could help him do something about that. Kevin had and has such a good heart, he was such an essentially fine person, that we let the real problem slide. We knew he was an addictive personality. But addictive personalities can deal with their problems, we thought. If they have all the support and love they need, they've got a good chance of doing that. Kevin had that from both of us, we thought, so we didn't reach farther down.

When Kevin finished high school, he enrolled at the University of Arkansas in Fayetteville. It was during his second year there that we began picking up signals that there was trouble. Kevin had started drinking. When we realized that, it startled us at first. I don't think Kevin ever had a beer in his life when he was living at home. Nobody in the family did any drinking to speak of. But we began to understand that now he was drinking a lot, not like binge drinking at college parties but real serious drinking. Some weekends he'd come home from school swaying into the house in an alcoholic daze.

Chapter 13

Joycelyn Elders, M.D.

Oliver and I both were at a loss for what to do. We didn't know if Kevin needed treatment or if this was something temporary that he was going to get a handle on. With him living up in Fayetteville it was difficult to tell exactly what was going on or how we could best help. Mainly we just worried and watched.

Strangely maybe, the anxiety I was feeling in my personal life at that time didn't seem to affect the research I was doing in the laboratory. There we were in the middle of tracking down what I thought might turn out to be a significant addition to our understanding of diabetes mellitus. I was still working hard on problems of growth and sexuality, but the majority of my time was now given over to treating children with diabetes.

Diabetes is by far the most common pediatric endocrine disease, and in the late seventies and early eighties diabetes research was exploding. We already knew a lot about the metabolism: how insulin works and what happens when there's an insufficiency. Now we were learning about insulin resistance. This was a whole other dimension of diabetes, which until then had been more or less a blank sheet. Often individuals who produced normal amounts of insulin suffered the same diabetic problems as people whose pancreases didn't work at all. Why was that? I had one little girl who came into the clinic with insulin levels of a thousand, when a hundred is high. Yet with all that insulin in her system, she still had diabetes. What was going on there?

Many researchers were looking at abnormalities in the insulin hormone. In my lab we were focusing on the process by which insulin passes from the bloodstream into the cell. In a certain category of cases, including my little thousand-insulin-level girl, normal insulin wasn't sticking to the cell wall and getting through to the inside. How did the receptor that was supposed to bind it to the cell normally work, and what was the nature of its disorders? There was a biochemical mystery going on here that just absorbed me.

On these diabetes studies I was collaborating with colleagues at various institutions around the country, including the University of Chicago, Joslin Clinic, and the National Institutes of Health. From time to time we met to coordinate our experiments and discuss our results. Since nobody had everything set up in one lab, we split the work according to who was best equipped to do it. That way things got done quickly. We learned fast and wrote up paper after paper. Some of our studies helped define the basic processes of insulin resistance.

Almost always diabetes is a disease that repays all the work you can put into it. It is fascinating. It is lethal. And if you treat it correctly, you get dramatic improvement. In almost all cases, if you do the right thing today, your patient will be well tomorrow. There's considerable satisfaction in that. In fact endocrine diseases as a group tend to be satisfying. Once you make a correct diagnosis, you get fast results. In that way endocrinology is a little like surgery. There's that same kind of quick-fix appeal to it.

The big difference is that endocrine diseases don't go away just because you've gotten your patient well. You can't fix it and forget it. Most other doctors spend the majority of their professional lives taking care of acute disease. But diabetes and the other endocrine diseases are chronic. Once you've got them, you've got them forever.

So endocrinologists are chronic disease specialists, which means they're always in for the long haul. When my urologist colleague John Redman and I would talk about surgical solutions for sexual abnormalities, my point of view always came from knowing that I was going to be caring for our patients from infancy right into adulthood or at least as long as I was in business. Even when I was out of doctoring, when I was director of public health, some of my long-term endocrine patients came to see me. They were used to my managing their cases, and sometimes I'd be taking a look at them right in the middle of policy meetings in the health department conference room. A surgeon can examine a problem, diagnose it, cut it out, patch it up, and that's it. But where endocrinologists shine is in how well they take care of their patients for the next twenty years.

That shapes your mentality. What also shapes it, especially when you concentrate on diabetes, is that to treat the disease effectively, you have to look at the patient's entire world. Diabetes affects everything a child does. It involves his family, his church, his school, and everyone else who's significantly associated with him. As a doctor you are not just dealing with a patient and his disease; you are dealing with the patient's whole living environment.

If a patient gets too much insulin, his blood sugar gets real low. He becomes hypoglycemic and has a reaction that may manifest as a seizure. If he gets too little, his acids build up, and he develops ketoacidosis and goes into a coma. Either condition can turn acute fast.

The only way to prevent these crises is through education. And you can't just educate the patient. You've got to educate everybody, as we found out, right down to the school bus drivers. One of the peak times when insulin acts is in the afternoon. In Arkansas, children from farm areas were often on the school bus going home at that time, and they weren't allowed to eat on the bus. So children were having reactions on the bus because they couldn't get their snacks in time. Teachers had to be educated, so if the child said he was hungry in the middle of the morning, they knew he had to eat or he might get hypoglycemic. The school had to know to prepare a special lunch, and the teacher had to know to keep candy in her desk. She also had to recognize the signs of a hypoglycemic reaction. Even the child's baby-sitter had to be aware and understand what to do.

Of course the family is the most critical. Parents need to be taught when to give more insulin, when to give food, when to see that the child exercises. And of course the child has to be as educated as you can possibly make him. In the hospital I always told my diabetic children, "I want you to get to where you can take care of your diabetes better than I can. Just as soon as you can do that, I'll let you go home."

In the early 1970s I got funding from the Public Health Service's Division of Maternal Child Health for a program we called Diabetes Education and Training. This program lasted five years and involved five hundred patients from all over Arkansas. In the course of it we developed a team concept of treatment, where each team would consist of a nurse, a social worker, and a nutritionist, as well as a doctor. On these teams the doctor wasn't necessarily the chief; the lead practitioner for any given case was the person who could deal most effectively with that individual child's particular problems. This wasn't a concept that doctors swallowed too easily then, though nowadays I think everyone understands its importance. Pretty much anybody can learn to juggle the insulin. It's the education part that really makes the difference.

Our goal was for patients and their parents to become knowledgeable enough to manage their own cases and confident they could do it. In time we got to be very proficient at that. The education we provided in that program reduced the incidence of hospitalization for diabetic ketoacidosis so much that Arkansas Medicaid started requiring that any child in the state who had been hospitalized twice for acute acidosis had to come see a pediatric endocrinologist, which at that time meant me. Otherwise Medicaid would not pay for a third hospitalization. We published the results of our team management approach in the Maternal Child Health publications, and the model was subsequently adopted for use throughout the country.

Though it didn't particularly occur to me at the time, all those years of working with diabetes and other endocrine diseases were teaching me a set of lessons about health in general. All that time I was doing research and teaching and seeing patients, I doubt I gave more than a few minutes of conscious thought to public policy. But looking back now, I can see that the work I was doing taught me a paradigm for health care that got itself ingrained in my thinking long before Bill Clinton hijacked me out of the university.

The pieces of that paradigm went something like this. If I took care of those diabetic children properly, I could practically eliminate emergency hospitalizations. In the longer run I could prevent complications of blindness, amputations, heart disease, kidney disease, stroke, and other drastic or fatal consequences. The key to this was in the word "prevent." All the resources you could put into prevention were repaid a thousand times over any way you wanted to figure it.

So prevention was the first piece of my paradigm, with education being the biggest part of prevention. The second was that problems tend to be systemic. They generally affect not just one isolated organ or function but a whole array of them. Pituitary problems usually mean adrenal, thyroid, sex, and, of course, growth problems. Insulin problems mean trouble for your heart, kidneys, liver, eyes, reproductive functions, and digestive system. It's all multiple. Almost anywhere you want to look, the foot bone's connected to the ankle bone. The next piece of the paradigm is that diseases tend to be social. Every pediatrician knows you have to treat the mom as well as the child. Every diabetes doctor knows it takes a whole range of people to make sure the child stays healthy. Finally, problems don't just disappear because you think you've figured out a cure. Really taking care of the child means constant, long-term, determined attention.

When I described this paradigm to one friend, she said, "All that talk about prevention and education and long term, no wonder you're a Democrat." She might have had something there. I think it's probably true that my politics developed along the vector of my profession. If I were a sociologist, I might want to spend some time just out of curiosity surveying endocrinologists to find out if their political persuasions are similar to mine.

When I became surgeon general—this was years after I had stopped being a diabetes specialist—my overriding goal was prevention, and my path to the goal was education. If you want to know the one thing I was about as a public health officer, that was it. In my speeches I used to say, "Ignorance is not bliss! We've tried ignorance; now let's try education!" The theme I hit on time after time after time was "If you don't educate people, you can't keep them healthy." Those were convictions I acquired in the diabetes clinic, long before I ever dreamed of becoming something different from a professor.

——

Girls with diabetes needed serious education not just about their diabetes but about sex. From the time I started doing endocrinology I was seeing enough pregnant teenage diabetics to drive me up a wall. Pregnancy can be a disaster for someone with diabetes. In *Steel Magnolias* Julia Roberts's character dies of it, an expectable outcome for someone who doesn't have her diabetes really well controlled. Not only does it put the mother's life in danger, but there's also a 50 percent increase in congenital abnormalities for babies of patients with uncontrolled diabetes.

In pregnancy, where the mother is feeding two rather than one, fuel consumption and fuel burning become especially crucial, which is precisely the function diabetes impacts on. When a woman gets pregnant, her blood volume goes up about 20 percent, to perfuse the placenta and feed the baby. Even healthy women tend to gain too much weight, retain salt and water, and get hypertensive. The additional blood volume puts extra stress on everything, including the circulatory system and kidneys.

In diabetics, who already have plenty of extra stress, the whole thing is just a mess. If treatment isn't good, you get cerebral edema overload and seizures. Plus, a good part of the girls we were dealing with were fifteen to seventeen years old, so their bodies weren't even completely prepared for pregnancy to begin with. They didn't have any business having babies yet under any circumstances. I'll never forget Ed Hughes's remark to a student who was a little confused about some aspect of the consequences of diabetes for pregnancy. After a couple of unsuccessful stabs at an explanation Ed said, "Dammit, son, teleologically the reason pregnancy is so bad for a diabetic mother is because God don't want her to have diabetic babies."

Which is fairly obvious when you are watching those babies in the pediatric intensive care unit. Infants of diabetic mothers tend to be very obese. In the old days they were called Campbell's soup babies because they looked like the fat cherubs that used to be on Campbell's soup labels. Often they are quite premature, yet their birth weight might be seven or eight pounds. For many years no one understood what was happening. When a baby that size got born, doctors assumed the timing of the gestation was just badly off for some reason. On the other hand, these seven-pound infants were behaving like two-pound preemies, which is what they really were.

What happens is that since the diabetic mother's blood coming across the placenta is high in sugar, the fetus compensates by producing large amounts of insulin. The oversupply of insulin makes the baby metabolize the sugars, and since the energy produced isn't needed, it's stored as fat. So the babies are born obese and hyperinsulin. They also tend to have hyaline membrane disease, underdeveloped lungs, low calcium, and hypoglycemia. The mortality is horrible.

To keep the girls I was treating from getting pregnant, I put them on Depo-Provera, which I was using for my precocious puberty cases. I told them, "I want you to have two good babies, and I'll decide when you can have them." They understood that they had to get their diabetes under perfect control before I was going to relent on this. And they were ready to go through whatever discipline was necessary so that when they were married and ready, they'd be able to carry through a pregnancy without endangering themselves or their infants. I'd talk to them and their parents about the necessity of birth control, and in all my years I never heard a single objection—just voices saying, "Yes, Dr. Elders," and heads nodding up and down in agreement.

I didn't want these girls dying, and I didn't want their babies dying. I had had enough of dying. But I confess that I had another motive too, which I didn't talk about with anyone at the time, except maybe Ed before he left. I knew that if I could get these teenage girls through until they were eighteen or nineteen and had high school diplomas instead of getting pregnant at fifteen and dropping out of ninth grade, their chances of making a decent life for themselves would go straight up. That was my own private public health policy I was following.

———

One girl who was in and out of the hospital from the time she was about eight was Nina, a little white girl from a town near Hot Springs. Nina's family situation was rough. Her mom and dad both were drinkers, and when I started seeing her, they were going through a divorce. From what I could tell, Nina's homelife was disintegrating, and every time there was some kind of event there, she ended up back in the hospital. The family crises were pretty frequent. At ten Nina was having to go around to bars to get her parents out and bring them home. Then after the divorce her mom left home, and her dad brought in a new girlfriend whom Nina had a hard time getting along with. Almost every other week Nina was in the hospital with diabetic ketoacidosis from not having taken her insulin. I told Oliver I wouldn't be surprised if one day she just turned up dead.

One Friday, when Nina was going through a really bad spell, she asked if she could come home with me for the weekend. She was about twelve at the time, and her parents' divorce had become final only a little while before. I didn't have to think too much about it. This wasn't the first time one of my patients who was going through troubles had asked, and one or two of them had come to stay for a bit. So I told Nina she could, and when I left the hospital that day, she came with me.

That was a good weekend for Nina. Kevin, who was three or four years older than she was, took her to the mall, and all in all, she seemed to have a good time. Over the next while, Nina came to stay several other weekends.

Having an extra in the house wasn't anything unusual. For

years we had been taking in one or another of Oliver's basketball players who might be having difficulties at home and needed a place to stay. Oliver was not just a coach to his boys; he was a role model and a personal counselor. If somebody didn't have a place to stay or something was happening in the family, Oliver invited him, and the boy came, sometimes for overnight or sometimes for a month. It wasn't even something we had to talk about. We just put another plate on the table, which became our term for it: just another plate on the table. Over the years we had so many visitors and strays that Stephen Kemp, one of my pediatric colleagues, started calling my house Elders' Arms.

So there was nothing unusual about having Nina around weekends. But then, when she got to be about fifteen, she asked if she could come live with us. What she wanted was for me to take her in permanently. Nina was still going through these bouts with her parents and still experiencing insulin crises that had her in the hospital a week or two at a stretch. I knew that she had been in and out of foster care situations and state facilities and that nothing had worked out for her. I thought that maybe she was beginning to doubt her own chances of surviving.

By now I had been taking care of Nina for seven or eight years, so we knew each other pretty well. And of course she had stayed with us and felt comfortable in the house. But when she asked this, I said, "Oh, Nina, I'm too old and tired for such a thing."

On the other hand, when this happened, Eric was a junior or senior in college already and Kevin had left for the university in Fayetteville. There were no children in the house anymore, and Oliver was usually out all day Saturday practicing. I was feeling a little lonesome, or at least that was how I interpreted it. What I was really doing was suffering from empty nest syndrome. So even though I might have told Nina I was too old and tired, in fact I was a setup for what she was asking. When I talked to Oliver about it, he said, "Well, Sug, if you think that that's what you want to do, then do it. All it is is another plate."

When I began looking into what it would take to have her stay with me, I learned that I would need to become a foster parent. That was already beyond what I had in mind. I wasn't interested in formalizing this in any way. I just wanted to take her in. But Nina kept after me, and meanwhile she was in the hospital again with nowhere really to go. So in the end I went out and started foster parent classes. Those took six weeks, and for the whole of that time we kept Nina in the hospital because she had nowhere else to go. Then we had to go to court to get her assigned to the department of human services, which then designated Oliver and me as legal guardians, all of this with the approval of Nina's parents. That still wasn't the end of it. Nina had no insurance of her own, and since she couldn't get onto my medical insurance for a year, we had to get her covered by Medicaid, a battle by itself.

Finally all these things were resolved. Oliver and I took her in and enrolled her at Northeast High. Everyone was pleased, especially Nina's parents. By this time her father had married again, though her mother was still having problems and was sometimes better, sometimes worse. But they knew that she had a stable home at least and that I'd be looking after her diabetes. We arranged it so that they could come get her whenever they wanted and that Nina could go home and visit whenever she wanted, which she used to do sometimes on weekends.

Nina went to tenth grade out of our house. But right from the start life with her wasn't easy. When she got to be sixteen, she started running away, and though she'd always come back, her school attendance was spotty. Pretty soon she was gone as much as she was there. She knew how upset I was about all this, but she didn't seem able to stop acting out the problems she had had for pretty much her whole life.

When she was seventeen, Nina quit school and got involved with a man who was several years older. Once she linked up with him, she left the house altogether, although many days she would come see me at the hospital. Most often she would also show up for the appointments I made for her to see a psychiatrist who was trying to help her work things through. Every so often someone would come up to Oliver on the street and say, "Hey, Coach. How you doin'? I saw your daughter the other day."

With her flaxen hair and blue eyes, Nina enjoyed telling people that Coach Elders was her daddy. Oliver would say, "I don't have a daughter." But Nina always knew she had a place to come back to.

Despite the people she was hanging around with, I thought that Nina had a good chance of making it. Although she wasn't living with me any longer, she went back to school and got her GED. Then she enrolled in nursing school. She was a bright girl, but her devils always seemed to be haunting her one way or another. Finally we heard she was getting into trouble with the law. By then she was probably nineteen and the only times we were seeing her were the holidays. On Christmas and Easter and July Fourth she would make sure to drop by and say hello.

———

We were upset by what was going on in Nina's life. And this was also the time we were doing some serious worrying about Kevin. But when I sat back and thought about it, in essence my life didn't seem a lot different from those of other medical school people. Like everyone else, I was doing my teaching and research and seeing patients, which was work I loved. And if there were any of my colleagues who didn't have their own private sorrows and worries, I wasn't aware of it. The only thing that was truly different about me was my skin. I had been the first black faculty member at Arkansas, and I was still the only black faculty member.

That might have made a difference in certain ways, like in the initial reactions some patients may have had to me or in the personal understanding I had about the lives of our poor black patients. But in essence my professional life wasn't visibly affected by race except in one way. Whether I wanted to be or not, I was an attraction, and neither the medical school nor the university ever forgot it. Every time they were recruiting somebody, from professors to deans, they always made sure the person got to meet me. If they had been recruiting a new president, that individual would have been brought down to my office first thing.

Often it was the recruits who took the initiative. People knew I was at Arkansas, and they wanted to come talk to me. And what they usually wanted to talk to me about was, How did they treat black people in this school? If they wanted to bring a black assistant professor with them, they'd want to know, would he get a fair shake down here?

My answer to that one was yes. I'd gotten a fair shake, and I felt that anybody they brought with them would too. From where I was standing, it looked like the university administrators were trying very hard on that front. They were reaching out to take more black students and trying to recruit black faculty, although they were in a rough competitive situation both ways. The cream of the black students was being skimmed off by places like Harvard and Stanford, tuition free, with offers that a state school couldn't begin to touch. As far as blacks in academic medicine were concerned, there just weren't that many around, so the demand was intense. If you were getting offers from Mass General and Johns Hopkins, you probably weren't going to give a lot of consideration to Arkansas. But that didn't mean the university wasn't trying. It was. So I was pretty well satisfied on that score, which made it easier being the one real visible black person there.

As far as my colleagues went, I'm sure a lot of heads turned when I came on as chief resident, but by now I was just another part of the scenery. No one treated me with either kid gloves or hostility, partly because I didn't treat anyone that way. People also knew that while I might be a good recruitment ad for the university, I was also being recruited myself. Over the years I was offered chairmanships at Morehouse and Meharry and Drew and Emory University. The NIH also asked me to come on as head of one of its major divisions, which any pediatric professor would have given her right arm for. But I never accepted any of them partly because I wasn't comfortable about giving up a big chunk of my research time to do administration but mostly because of the understanding Oliver and I had about our careers.

Oliver was coaching at Hall High, where he had moved after

Horace Mann. At Hall he won seven conference titles, three state divisional championships, and two overall state championships. He was universally acknowledged to be the state's leading high school coach. That was considerable fame in a place as crazy about basketball as Arkansas, and from time to time he got coaching offers from colleges. Of course, if you really want to pursue a big-time coaching career in basketball, you first have to get college-level experience. You don't just get picked out of the high school ranks by an Indiana or a UCLA. So the college offers Oliver got tended to be from smaller schools. But he never took them because the four-year colleges were mostly in small communities. If we moved to one of those places, I wouldn't have had a job except if maybe I wanted to be the school doctor.

The offers I was getting would have put Oliver in more or less the same situation. The end result was that neither of us was willing to move unless the other one could also get a job that made sense. So number one, whoever wanted one of us was going to have to want the other. Number two was that we both were really happy where we were, so any incentive to pull up roots would have had to be more than just normally persuasive. We didn't like the idea of picking ourselves up and moving.

Actually I was getting a full share of professional satisfaction without a chairmanship. As the number of papers I wrote and presentations I gave mounted, I found myself being included in some elevated circles. I was selected for the Society for Pediatric Research, which has 450 members out of about 40,000 practicing pediatricians. I became a member of the Lawton Wilkens Pediatric Endocrine Society, and eventually I was elected president of the Southern Society for Pediatric Research.

Starting in the late seventies, I was also asked to serve on several NIH "study sections." These are the committees that review grant proposals and make awards, so the members exert a powerful influence on the direction of American research. At one time or another I was on the maternal/child health section, the human embryology and development section, and the rural health advisory committee, each of which met four times a year outside Washington.

That was just ideal. Pat was living in Silver Spring, Maryland, with her husband, Sidney, and their three children, so on my trips to the NIH I got to stay over and visit with her and the family. By then Pat was teaching linguistics at Howard and making frequent trips to Africa to trace the origins of the folktales and customs she was finding on the Sea Islands. Together with the photographer Jeanie Ashe, Arthur Ashe's wife, she did a big Sea Island story for *National Geographic,* and she was busy preparing her book *When Roots Die,* about the lives and literature of the islands' Gullah people.

I loved those trips to Washington, and I loved her children, Brianne and Beenie and Antonia, all of whom used to stay with us during the summer, which was when Pat made her field trips. The kids always enjoyed coming down to Arkansas, where they got to spend time not just with Oliver and me but down on the farm with their grandma and grandpa. I had taken care of Pat for the first few years of her life, then Oliver and I had kept her while she was in nursing school, so we had been kind of like surrogate parents. Now I was getting to know Pat as an adult, just as I had gotten to know Bernard again. With that, and with her children coming to us, I felt like we were reintegrating the family.

In 1978, around the same time I began serving on the NIH study sections, I also got involved in writing up the board certification examinations for pediatric endocrinologists. Up till then pediatric endocrinology was not a formal medical specialty. When I started, I doubt there were more than fifteen or twenty of us in the country, though now there must be a couple of thousand.

When pressure began to grow to establish pediatric endocrinology as a recognized subspecialty, a small group of pediatricians was picked to take the general endocrinology boards. This group then devised questions for a pediatric board certification, and about fifteen of us took that first exam, including Ed Hughes, who by that time had moved to Southern Alabama University to help start up its new medical school, and me. Ed says I did better than he did, but I don't remember that, and it doesn't sound likely. Anyway, since nobody was grandfathered in, Ed and I were among the first board-certified pediatric endocrinologists, after which a group of us developed the next board exams. That was a labor-intensive process. It included field tests and questions to determine the appropriate level of difficulty and intensive review. Over a period of years we defined the discipline.

———

At some point while all this was going on, a very peculiar thing happened to me. I lost the consciousness of being black. One day in the department of public health when I was director, I overheard my deputy, Tom Butler, telling someone, "She doesn't know if she's white or black. She doesn't care about it." Tom was wrong. I knew for sure what I was, and I cared. But somewhere along the line it just stopped making any difference.

I can't put my finger on exactly when that happened. I'm sure it was gradual. When I was growing up, the one thing you were conscious of even when you were asleep was what color you were. That was in the thirties and forties, when segregation was so much a way of life you never thought of anything different. Whites were up here and blacks were down here, and that was the way it was. You didn't go to church or school or college with white folks; you didn't compete against them in athletics. In large chunks of your life you didn't interact with them at all. So it wasn't that you went around feeling inferior all day long. It wasn't near you all the time. But there was no doubt about it, you did feel inferior.

I did, even though our own experience with the white people we knew in our community was generally good. I did, even right down to admiring their beautiful hair. You grow up in apartheid, that's what gets ingrained in you a thousand different ways. I believed they were probably better than we were. Why else would Mama say, "You've got to be as good as whites. You want to get somewhere, you got to be *better* than whites"? For Mama and for our teachers, it wasn't enough just to be a good black person; you had to be good enough to be as good as the best white person. What that meant was that they were up there on a different level to start with. We just thought that was natural.

Somewhere or other I lost that feeling of inferiority. Maybe going to school with white kids in California and doing well there had something to do with it, or maybe my record at Howard County Training School, or my college performance. Whatever it was, when I joined the Army, I don't remember feeling inferior in any way to the seventeen young women I went through physical therapy school with. But though we were all friends and I might not have felt inferior, I was still intensely aware that they were white and I was black. I thought about that all the time.

Medical school, where I was one of three black students, was the same. At Minnesota I was *the* black intern; then back in Arkansas I was the black resident. I was even the *first* black resident. Even when I was chief resident, I still considered myself the black chief resident. Actually I thought of myself as the *black female* chief resident because my consciousness had been raised by then. I was very proud of me. I was proud of where I was, and I was proud of who I was. I was every bit as aware of my blackness as I had been back down in Schaal.

But later on there came some moment when I no longer thought of myself as Joycelyn Elders the black doctor, or Joycelyn Elders the woman doctor, or Joycelyn Elders the this or the that. I was just plain Dr. Elders. That was a moment I was aware of only in retrospect. I don't know when I slid into that new identity. I do know when I was at the health department, I never once thought of myself as the black health director. So to that extent I guess Tom was right.

For me the important question isn't when but how. What is it that enables you to get loose from that racial fixation, to get out from under the constant awareness of it? In my case I think it had to do with being a scientist, though I think maybe you could substitute almost any other profession for science. Somewhere in my development as a scientist and a doctor, my profession began to take hold of the way I thought about myself.

When my papers were published in scientific journals they were not signed "Joycelyn Elders, M.D., Black Woman," just "Joycelyn Elders, M.D." And when scientists in New York or California or Europe read them, they judged them on the basis of their cogency and persuasiveness, nothing else. Before I left the university, I published almost 150 papers. In each one of those I was measured against the standards of my peers. That will change you. That was a career's worth of experience at seeing myself through the eyes of my profession.

My most powerful moment of this kind was given to me by one of my students, a young white male who worked in my lab from the time he was in college right up through med school. I had taught him and guided him. I had torn his work down again and again and watched him build it back up to the point where he produced a significant study of the effect of glucocorticoids on growth.

That was an important piece of research, and it still is, after many years. And when he presented it to the Society for Pediatric Research, I was the only black person in the auditorium. Well, this boy's work was beautiful, and his presentation was beautiful. I felt an overwhelming pride that he was my student and I was his teacher. I hadn't become any less black or female than I ever had been. But this was my profession telling me loud and clear what standards mattered here.

That voice stayed in my head. Later, when I moved into public life, it was my strength and, from a certain point of view, also my weakness. I had a strong tendency not to be that careful about the political implications of what I did. Instead I tried to understand what was correct scientifically and do that. What was right and made sense had no racial or gender color. Most of all, it had no political color. For a scientist that approach was as noncontroversial as you could get. For a public servant it had some drawbacks.

Chapter 14

In the Midst of Life

❧

By his third year at the university Kevin's drinking had got to the point where he stopped going to classes. We didn't know. When he came home at the end of the first semester that year, he didn't say anything about that. He also didn't tell us that because he wasn't going to classes, his grades were so bad that he had flunked out of school. He was so desperate to keep it a secret that when the new semester began, he drove back up to Fayetteville as if nothing were wrong. But when he was told he had to move out of the dorm, we found out. There was no alternative for him but to come back to Little Rock.

Once he was at home, Kevin started working for Oliver on our rental properties. My idea was that he should work for a while and get his bearings, without any pressure on him. Then, once he felt better, I'd see what I could do about getting him enrolled at Philander Smith so he could finish college.

But our hopefulness didn't last long. One day he came home with a DWI ticket, driving while intoxicated. Then we found out this was his second offense, which meant an automatic license suspension. Without a car the property job disappeared. But Kevin went to the alcohol education classes, and when the suspension was up, he got back behind the wheel.

When I went over to Philander Smith to talk to them about

Kevin, they were very receptive. Ordinarily they would make someone who had flunked out wait a year before considering him, but after I explained the situation, they decided to take a chance. So that summer Kevin began school again. Classes at Philander Smith went all right. Kevin was still drinking on occasion, but it seemed to us that he had it under control. At least he wasn't letting it keep him from passing his courses. By then Oliver and I were thankful for anything we could get.

By Kevin's last semester, though, things had got considerably worse. Checks started bouncing in our property accounts, and when we looked at it, it turned out that he was using the money. When we asked what he needed it for, he came out and told us. He was spending it on alcohol and drugs.

I think that up to that point Oliver and I felt that this was something that could be cleared up or at least lived with. We understood that Kevin had a drinking problem, but that didn't necessarily mean he was an alcoholic. He was functioning, going to school and working. As long as he was doing that and wrestling with it so it wasn't controlling his life, that was as much as we thought we could ask for. But now we understood that Kevin's problems were at a different level from what we had believed. And it wasn't just alcohol. This was the first we learned that drugs were in the picture too. Neither of us was dealing all that well even with Kevin's drinking. This new development sent shivers through us.

We knew we had to get Kevin into treatment. But it's obvious to me, looking back, that we still didn't have a good understanding of how deep this problem went. I got the name of a good treatment center, and when we called, they wanted us to bring him down that day. But there were only two weeks to go in the semester, and we thought it would be a better idea to let him finish up, then go in after that.

Kevin was amenable to anything we decided. He also assured us he could stay clean until he went in. He felt positive that once he got detoxified, he would be all right. So we pulled back and let him finish. Then we took him down.

Two weeks later, on New Year's Day, we got a call from the

center. The previous night Kevin had sneaked out and gotten some drugs for himself and a couple of other patients. The center was putting him out immediately; we should come get him. The staff recommended another center that they felt would be better equipped to handle him. They even talked about having him arrested if we didn't get him into another program without any delay. On our way to pick him up neither Oliver nor I spoke. Oliver drove. I sat there remembering how easy I had had it when Kevin was young, how I used to be so satisfied that he and Eric were never any trouble—too satisfied, I was thinking as we drove down to get him. So self-satisfied I couldn't see whatever it was that was troubling him so badly.

We ended up taking Kevin to a rehabilitation program in Monroe, Louisiana, not far from Grambling College. This new place seemed to have a positive effect. He completed the live-in requirement without any problem, then enrolled at Grambling and went in for treatment each evening as an outpatient while he was studying. From what we could tell, the program was working. Kevin's grades were good, and he didn't miss a single one of his nightly sessions. When we went down to see him, he seemed cheerful and optimistic about the progress he was making. By this time we didn't know what to think, but all the signs looked good, and we were trying our hardest to believe that the worst was behind him.

Kevin finished out the semester at Grambling, then went back to Philander Smith to complete his bachelor's in business administration. Although we tried not to, we found ourselves watching him like a hawk, looking for any telltale signs of drinking or drug use, meanwhile praying as hard as we could that we wouldn't find any. Every day we didn't was another day of relief. We were even happier when Kevin decided to enroll in the M.B.A. program at Grambling. It seemed to us that he was making an all-out effort and that maybe this time he truly had gotten himself clean. I felt really good that things were working out, the first time in ages I didn't feel that maybe I was trying to convince myself of something that might not be true.

Every addict's loved ones learn hard lessons, but it often takes time. Oliver and I understood we still had a lot of learning in front of us when we got a call one day from a police station in some town in northwestern Arkansas. Kevin was on the phone. He had just been arrested for driving while intoxicated.

In Arkansas, a third DWI means loss of license and six months in jail. Up in that part of the state we knew we couldn't look for any kind of consideration either. But the judge did something unexpected. He dismissed the court and had Kevin, Oliver, and me come back in his office, where he sat us down and talked to us for a long time. When he got finished, he gave Kevin his license back. "You can go down there to Grambling," he said (of course we had told him that Kevin was about to start graduate school). "I'm going to let you go on down there. But you are going to have to bring your grades up here to me every semester, personally. And I'm promising you right now, if you ever get anything less than a B, I'm going to throw you in jail so fast your head will spin. You understand that? One C and you are in jail!"

Kevin had never done really well in school, ever. He was bright, but he just didn't seem to be a good student, even though I always thought that maybe he was a better student than anybody gave him credit for. I got that idea one semester in junior high school when we experimented with paying him for his grades and he made all As and Bs. But other than that he had never done especially well, until that master's program at Grambling with the judge's threats hanging over his head. Whether that judge scared Kevin to death or what, I don't know, but he got the best grades of his life and he finished that M.B.A. program with flying colors.

After that we didn't hear anything more about either alcohol or drugs. The big problem was finding a job, which was tough at that time in Arkansas, even with an M.B.A. But eventually that worked out too. Kevin got a position at the Johnson & Johnson plant in North Little Rock as a products manager, which paid well and was a good fit for his skills. Before long he had forty-five people working for him, and he was living by himself in one of our rental houses. It looked for all the world as if he had fought his battles and finally gotten the upper hand.

———

Arkansas is often described as a small southern state, which is true. You get an idea of how small from Little Rock, the capital and largest city, which is six exits on the freeway and has a population of 150,000. What that means is that everybody knows everybody else, especially in circles like business, politics, football, and the academic world. The reason there aren't any secrets in Arkansas is that the most visible people all call each other by first name and have lunch together. Somebody or other always knows who did what, and after that most of the rest of them know it too. How deals go down, political or business or whatever, is something discussed over coffee. In a big state it would be private information, but in a small state you say, "Gee, how did they put that together?" and somebody or other is going to tell you.

Probably the first person I met from the political sphere was Betty Bumpers, the wife of Dale Bumpers, who was governor from 1970 to 1974 and has been a U.S. senator since then. Dale Bumpers always fought hard for public health, especially childhood immunization, which was Betty's special interest. He used to say that if he didn't, Betty wouldn't let him come home at night.

I believe that could actually have been true, since I had firsthand experience of Betty Bumpers's commitment to getting children vaccinated. Her immunization drives were more like crusades. She organized everybody in the state. She would call us up at the medical school and say, "Saturday, November seventeenth, is going to be a major immunization drive. I'm getting everybody out this time. I've got the National Guard setting up sites and the police going door to door and the Army giving me nurses. It's scheduled to run from twelve to six, and the Kiwanis is providing transportation. Now, I need everybody in your department to help give shots, and here's where I want them to be." And on November 17 every member of the pediatric faculty who wasn't on emergency call or something, including me, was standing in an armory or a fire station giving shots all afternoon. Once Betty Bumpers got three hundred thousand children vaccinated against polio in a single day.

That was how I met Betty Bumpers. Then Dale Bumpers appointed me to be on his Commission on the Status of Women, so I met him too, although I can't say we knew each other well. Once, years later, when I was health director, I was testifying in front of a Senate committee Bumpers was on, and he said, "My goodness, Dr. Elders, where were you when I lived in Arkansas?"

So I said, "Senator, when you were governor, you appointed me to your Commission on the Status of Women," and he said, "Well, all right, I knew I had good sense." Dale Bumpers has always been an extremely delightful person with a real good sense of humor.

One Arkansas mover and shaker Bumpers didn't like much was Witt Stephens, whom I also met when I was a young professor. Mr. Witt, as everyone called him, was the most powerful man in the state hands down. He had started off in the Depression selling sundries like Bibles and condoms, then afterward started up a little brokerage business that he eventually built into a family company that became the biggest investment firm west of the Mississippi. The reason Dale Bumpers didn't like him was that Mr. Witt was big in natural gas, among other things; he was the president and a major stockholder in ArkLa, the Arkansas Louisiana Gas Company. As a young country lawyer in western Arkansas Dale Bumpers used to go around suing Mr. Witt and the other big players on behalf of small leaseholders who were being taken advantage of.

Shortly after I had joined the faculty at the medical school, a political friend of mine who was trying to run for office took me up to meet Mr. Witt. He had invited us to lunch at his office, which was something he was famous for. He had a full-service kitchen up there and gave the kind of Arkansas country lunches that made you think of pioneering days, with smoked hams and

turkeys and ribs and black-eyed peas and corn bread and whatever else you might want to imagine. "Why don't y'all come on
up so we can break bread together?" he'd rumble in a kind of
low, hoarse voice that he liked to modulate for effect. One veteran reporter I knew used to have lunch with him on occasion
and in later years liked to tell stories of what would happen
while they ate. During the meal someone would come in and
murmur something like "They want to know if we'll sell the
bonds now," and Mr. Witt would stage-whisper back, "Not yet."
Later the same person would come back in, and Mr. Witt would
say, "Okay, now." A minute later he'd wipe his chin and smile.
"You know," he'd say, "I just made thirty million dollars." All
without missing a mouthful.

Mr. Witt was a big man, fat and jolly, who puffed on a big
cigar and looked like somebody's grandfather. When I met him,
he told me he'd been following what I was doing; he knew all
about it. He knew that I had been chief resident; he knew about
my NIH fellowship. He'd been keeping an eye on me. Saying
it that way sounds slightly ominous, but there wasn't the least
bit of discomfort in the way he put it. He just gave you the idea
that he knew everything that went on in the state because it was
his natural business to know it, because he was the godfather.
The next time we met was after I was inducted into the Society
for Pediatric Research. When that happened, he invited me up
again to congratulate me, then wrote me a warm personal letter.
I wasn't the only academic who got that treatment from him.
Mr. Witt was so attuned that he even kept track of who was
doing what at the university.

One of Mr. Witt's brightest protégés, whom I also knew, was
Sheffield Nelson. Sheffield started off as a shining young star in
Mr. Witt's firmament; Mr. Witt made him president of the
ArkLa Gas Company when he was only thirty-three. But things
subsequently happened that turned them into bitterest enemies,
and it was their enmity that in a way was ultimately responsible
for triggering the Whitewater mess.

I first met Sheffield even before he became president of
ArkLa, when he was just one of Mr. Witt's boys. Sheffield had

been a star student and political leader at Arkansas State Teachers College after coming out of a childhood in rice-growing country that was as hard as my own. Mr. Witt noticed him and gave him a job at ArkLa when he graduated, then eventually handed the presidency over to him when he himself decided to step down.

What happened after that I heard about the same as everyone else in Arkansas did. It was in the courts for years. The outlines are that after he stepped down, Mr. Witt wanted ArkLa to carry gas from his fields in western Arkansas to the east through its pipeline, which was the only way to get it out of there. But Sheffield, who was president now, refused to do it, despite the fact that he owed his job to Mr. Witt. He thought it was a bad deal for the Arkansas ratepayers. The Stephens family and other gas producers in western Arkansas had no alternative but to sell their gas to ArkLa at ArkLa's prices, since there was no way for them to get the gas out to other buyers, and Sheffield didn't see any reason to give up his purchase monopoly.

Among the things Witt Stephens was famous for was his feelings about the sanctity of gratitude. Everybody in Arkansas had heard stories about how if someone had shown some tiny kindness to Witt's daddy half a century ago and Witt heard that this person's son was having trouble, he'd find some way to help that son. Mr. Witt had his faults, but nobody ever accused him of not having a heart as big as a barn when it came to being grateful. Mr. Witt was also known as the forgiving type. But what Sheffield Nelson did to him on that pipeline deal was such an affront to his dearest-held values that it could never be forgiven.

In the middle of the court fights between Sheffield and the Stephens family, *The New York Times* published an article about some Stephens gas-dealing shenanigans that embarrassed Mr. Witt considerably. Everybody was wondering where the *Times* had gotten its information from, and eventually it came out that Sheffield Nelson was the main source for that story. Later the Stephenses got back by leaking their own story to the *Times* about a giant sweetheart deal Sheffield had made as head of ArkLa with Jerry Jones, who came out of it with so much money that he went off and bought the Dallas Cowboys. That same story broke again in the *Arkansas Gazette* in even more damaging form when Sheffield was running for governor in 1990. Word was that the Stephenses were behind that too.

That happened during the Republican primary, when Sheffield was running against one of the Stephenses' political allies. Sheffield had been a lifelong liberal Democrat, but he got so tired of waiting for Bill Clinton to stop being governor and give him a turn that he switched over to Republican. It didn't help him, though. He won the Republican primary in 1990, but the Jerry Jones scandal really hit him hard, and it refused to go away during his race against Clinton. It seemed like it was front-page news for months.

That was a really nasty election. Not only was Sheffield killed by the Jerry Jones scandal, but he also got hit on the head by allegations he was a womanizer. Worse was how angry he was at Clinton for even running. Everybody had thought Clinton was going to run for President in 1988. When he decided not to, it was at the last moment and surprised even his friends. After Dukakis lost to George Bush, it was such a sure bet that Clinton would run in 1992 that it became an issue in the 1990 governor's race as to whether he was just looking for temporary employment or did he really mean to be a full-time governor.

Sheffield Nelson kept badgering him on that, asking did he intend to finish out his term if he was elected, and Clinton kept finessing the answer, saying things like "I have no present plans to run." Finally Sheffield cornered him during one television debate, and Clinton said something that sounded pretty definite about serving it out. In the end Clinton just destroyed Sheffield. I think Clinton might have taken every county in Arkansas. Sheffield came out of that race humiliated by the vote and with his name dragged through the mud by scandal. To stoke up his fury even more, Clinton of course started his run for President scarcely a year later.

Those who know him say that afterward Sheffield was a bitter, bitter man. Bill Clinton became his most hated enemy. I don't care if you're talking about it's raining; somehow Clinton made this drop fall over here on Sheffield's head. All the old-time political observers down here were watching to see what kind of vindictiveness was going to come out of it.

They didn't have to wait all that long. Jeff Gerth, the *New York Times* reporter who broke the Whitewater case nationally, was the same one Sheffield had given the Stephens gas chicanery story to years back. Sheffield gave him Whitewater too, although Whitewater was nothing new in Arkansas. Clinton's investment in that deal had been used against him in one of his early races for governor, though it never came to anything. It's an open secret in Little Rock that not only is Sheffield the source for a lot of the Whitewater information but also that he was the one who persuaded Jim McDougal to talk to Gerth. Sheffield has been a big help to Al D'Amato's committee, though of course the Republicans have gone overboard to keep his name out of the news.

I got to really know Sheffield long before his anger at Clinton blossomed. When he was still president of ArkLa, he asked if I would be on the board of the Little Rock Chamber of Commerce. I picked up the phone one day in my office at the medical school, and a voice said, "Dr. Elders, this is Sheffield Nelson."

I was so astounded that this man who was one of the most important business leaders in the state was making his own call instead of having a secretary do it that I just said, "Yes, sir."

"I'm going to be president of the Chamber of Commerce this year," the voice said, "and I want more diversity. I wanted to know if you would serve on the board."

I agreed. I was assigned to work on the education committee, and I developed a very high regard for Sheffield's ability to run a meeting, get people working together, and get involved with what was going on in the community.

I was so impressed that when I became health director, I wanted to appoint Sheffield to head our long-range planning committee. This was in the period before the 1990 gubernatorial election, when it was already clear he was going to run. I thought Sheffield would be absolutely the smartest, most talented person I could get. But I also knew he'd try to use the position as a springboard for his governor's race, which didn't take much figuring out since he made no bones about it. So I talked it over with Governor Clinton first, and he said if I wanted to appoint him, that would be just fine. He thought Sheffield would do a real good job.

He did too. He chose the top people available for that committee, he organized them, and he made them work like dogs. He promised me he would be done with it by the end of December, and at the end of December he handed me a wonderful document that spelled out Arkansas's long-term health needs and how we should go about fulfilling them. That report addressed subjects like school-based clinics and health education in schools, including sex education, teenage pregnancy, condom distribution—all the big topics. When he handed it to me, he made sure to have all his public relations people, the TV and newspaper people, and everybody else he could think of right there to document the handing over.

Bill Clinton himself I first met when he appointed me to the Arkansas Industrial Development Commission; that was before Bernard died. He made the appointment, but it was actually Hillary who approached me about it. She called me up and said, "You know, industrial development is the most important issue Bill wants to take on this session, to try to build up our economy. We really feel that you could contribute to that, and it would mean a lot to us if you would do it." Specifically they wanted me to work on health issues related to industrial development, which was a fairly limited area. But on that commission you met all the big guns in Arkansas business, CEOs and bank presidents and so on. That was probably the first time I really felt my circle was expanding beyond the medical school.

After that I got to know Hillary fairly well, though we never became social friends. She was active in various women's organizations and events, and I had been on the Commission on the Status of Women and the Child Care Board and the Panel of American Women and other things. So our paths crossed now and then, even though I was never as active as I would have liked. I was so busy trying to combine my work with being a wife and mother that I just didn't have much time left over, which I regretted. We were also both in the Willow Institute, which was established to help develop young leaders for Arkansas.

What especially impressed me about Hillary was the work she did for us when I became health director. I often asked her to be honorary cochair of some panel or commission, which she would always do. But she wouldn't just lend her name. If she took something on, she got involved in it. She really wanted to know why we were having those particular problems the panel had been set up to address; then she dug her teeth into the issue and worked on it. There was no superficiality about Hillary Clinton. She wasn't an armchair do-gooder. She knew what her talents were, and she put them to use. She would decide what was the hardest problem Bill had, and she would take it on. I respected her as a woman and a wife for that. There was no question that we all thought she was extremely able.

———

In 1986 Chester came back to Arkansas to become pastor at Little Rock's Hunter United Methodist. Before that Chester had been doing some remarkable things. For many years he had been on the board of the Methodists' Global Ministries, spending part of his time out in the fields with migrant farm workers and supporting leaders like César Chavez. I'm not sure how many other religious workers could have understood the migrants' problems like Chester did. He knew them from the inside out. He had lived them personally.

Actually it was remarkable that Chester did any of the things he did. Other than Bernard, who had left home early, Chester was the one child who almost got away from Mama's compulsion to get everyone educated. She was just so busy with the farm and taking care of everyone that his reading almost slipped through the cracks. One time, when I was home visiting and Chester was in seventh grade, Mama was helping him with some math problem. But right in the middle she got distracted by someone else and said, "Chester, I don't have time for this. I've got to work with these little ones." When Chester started sniffling, Mama said, "Well, you just read while I'm doing this." And he started sounding things out, trying to pronounce letters.

Mama stared at him, stunned. She hadn't realized. She listened for a moment with her eyes open wide, then said half to herself, "Oh, my Lord, this child can't read!" Then she said, "Tomorrow at school you bring me back a primer." The next evening Mama started Chester on the primer and gradually moved him up until he learned to read enough so he could get to work by himself on the Bible.

Like Bernard, Chester went into the Army and became a paratrooper. Afterward he went to school at Baker University in Kansas, where he studied religion and philosophy, and somewhere along the line he realized he was called to the church. After college he enrolled in Gammon Theological Seminary, where he graduated with a master's in divinity and was ordained a minister by the United Methodists. Even that didn't satisfy his love of learning, and he later completed all his course work for a doctorate at Drew University.

I must say that Chester surprised me some when he decided on the ministry. It wasn't that he lacked faith or anything like that, but the idea of Chester as a minister had just never occurred to me. He was my rambunctious, roughhousing little brother. I would have guessed he'd go into farming, which he was very good at. He understood crops, and he was a nonstop worker. He had a large supply of dogged determination, which is the main ingredient a farmer needs. So having him be a minister took a little getting used to.

When Chester called from New York to tell me about his assignment in Little Rock, I felt the world had just got three shades brighter. I was so glad he was coming back. Of course I was proud of what he had done with his life since he left home, but my memories of past times with Chester were truly vivid. When he was a baby, I had held him on my lap the whole long way out to California by train, and once we were out there, he had been mine to take care of. It's Chester's face I remember best from the time the family picked early cotton to get me the bus ticket up to Philander Smith, and those words—"Do we have enough yet?"—that came out of his five-year-old mouth after he had been slaving for two days straight had carved themselves on my brain permanently.

For whatever reason, Chester had always got a lot of my attention when I used to visit home from medical school. As likely as not we'd end up working together out in the fields, or he'd corral me into taking him somewhere in my car. During one winter visit he had pneumonia, and Mama had had him cooped up inside for days. When she went out somewhere, I wrapped him in a couple of blankets and took him fishing. I thought it would be okay, and anyway, I was the one who was in medical school. When Mama came back, she was so furious I thought she was going to grab a switch and tan my legs.

All this is a long way of saying how I felt about Chester's coming back to Arkansas, which he did in July 1986. We helped him unload and get moved into the Hunter Methodist parsonage, and that night I fell asleep tired and happy. The next thing I knew the telephone was ringing on my night table, dragging me out of sleep. When I finally groped around for it and said hello, it was Sidney, Pat's husband, on the phone. "Mint," he said (he called me Mint, the same as my dad and Pat did), "I'm down here in South Carolina. I'm calling to tell you that Pat just died."

By now Oliver was up asking what was wrong. "Sidney," I said, "what in the world are you talking about?"

"She was in a car accident on the islands," Sidney was saying. "Brie was with her. Brie's okay, but Pat had a head injury. They had her on a respirator for a while, but the doctor said she was brain dead, and they've taken her off. Don't worry about Brie; she's okay. I'll call your parents and tell them. Let me do that."

A million thoughts were running through my head. Of course you don't comprehend these things at first; you're in shock. Okay, I was thinking, Pat's gone. Now, who's going to take care of her children? Sidney had a busy job at the Environmental Protection Agency, and I didn't know if he'd feel up to it. Besides, Pat had told me more than once that if anything ever happened to her, she wanted me to raise them, not that you ever think that something actually will happen. Besides, the girls had stayed with us so much, it'd be natural for them to come down and be our children. I think I was deciding on this issue even before I got out of bed to make coffee and try to calm myself down. Sidney will probably be grateful for it, I thought. Oliver loves them, and the girls will have a good life down here. So that's settled. Now, what else have I got to do?

It turned out that Pat had left instructions that she wanted to be cremated. She wanted her ashes spread over the fields where she used to work as a child. I think that was a shock for all of us when we heard about it. Cremation isn't a custom that has taken hold in the southern black community, so the idea seemed foreign and strange. But she had been very clear, and although Sidney wasn't happy about it either, he carried out her wishes.

Pat was cremated in South Carolina and first there was a memorial service in Washington at Howard University, which I went to with Chester. Then Sidney brought her ashes down to Schaal for committal to the earth. The funeral ceremony was held at our old Tabernacle Methodist, with Chester conducting. He kept saying beforehand, "You know, I came back down here to be with Mama and Daddy in their last years so I could bury them, and now the first thing that happens is that I've got to bury Pat." It was now a week since Pat's death, but none of us could believe it yet.

Chester gave the eulogy. Then we all walked out toward this big open hayfield that had been in our family since my grandfather's time, hundreds of people, grieving, Mama and Daddy and all our relations and friends down there, Eric and Kevin, some of Pat's close colleagues from up at Howard, Sidney and the girls holding one another's hands. Phillip had arranged for someone with a small airplane to fly over and scatter the ashes, and while we were walking toward the field, we heard the plane coming. As he flew low across the land, the plane gave out a cloud of orange smoke to show that Pat's ashes were released. Then, as the smoke hung there and started to dissipate, Chester spoke the words of committal. "In the midst of life, we are in death." Chester's strong voice was breaking, like our hearts were. "For all that Pat has given us to make us what we are/ For that part of Pat that lives and grows in each of us/And for Pat's life that in Your love will never end, we give You thanks/ As now we offer Pat back into Your arms."

———

While I was in Washington, I had asked Sidney if he wanted me to take the children back with me. He said no, he thought the family ought to be together. That was fine, but then, after we got home and the funeral was over, I talked to him seriously about the future. Antonia was thirteen, and Beenie was eleven, but little Brie was only two or three, barely more than a toddler. It was hard for me to see how Sidney would be able to manage with the three of them. Oliver and I could give them a loving home as long as necessary, at least until he was able to get his life together and felt up to taking them. The schools where we lived were good; they would be near their grandma and grandpa and other relatives. Frankly I felt it would be better for them. But Sidney had thought about it already, and he had made up his mind that he wanted his family to stay with him. I asked if he wanted me at least to keep Brie, and he told me no.

I had watched Sidney take care of the girls when I used to visit them in Washington. I had seen him get up in the morning to fix their breakfasts or get them ready for church on Sunday or take them out fishing with him. But I had real misgivings, especially about Brie. I worried a lot about her. But from the first Sidney became a superdad. When I went up to Washington on visits, I couldn't find a thing to complain about. Now, ten years after Pat's death, they have all grown into wonderful young people. Antonia went into the insurance business and has become a regional manager at a very young age, Beenie's a junior at Howard, and Brie is going into ninth grade. She's a wonderful basketball player, and her daddy runs around and takes her to all the games. She has him totally wrapped around her finger. I don't know if Sidney sees her like I do. But to me Brie is getting to look more and more like Pat all the time.

Chapter 15

But for the Grace of God

❦

Pat's death made 1986 a dreadful year. It wasn't even that happy a time for me at the medical school. After Ted Panos's death of a heart attack back in 1965, the pediatric chairmanship had never really settled down too well. Ed Hughes had been acting chairman before he left for West Virginia; then another chairman came in who was an excellent physician but who had a penchant for confrontation that aggravated a lot of people around the school, including the dean. He hung on for a long time, but he never had what you would call an easy tenure. When he was finally forced out, one common reaction was surprise that it had taken so long to do it.

Of the people they started looking at to fill the job, the leading candidate was Bob Fiser. Bob was a local Arkansas boy who had been a couple of years behind me in the medical school, then had gone out to California. I had brought him back from UCLA myself a few years earlier, hiring him to join me in pediatric endocrinology. Bob had always been a natural-born political animal, and we all knew he'd be a prime contender once the current chairman finally upset the dean one time too many.

Then, just at the point when he seemed on the verge of anointing Bob successor, the dean called me into his office to ask what would I think about taking the chairmanship myself.

This was on a Friday afternoon. Would I give it some consideration over the weekend, he said, then come see him first thing on Monday?

I had not been in the running for the chairmanship, so the idea wasn't something I had given any thought to. I had never been attracted much to administration, and this would mean managing people who had been my friends and colleagues forever. Well, I thought, that would be disagreeable several different ways; I'd for sure never take that on. But then I thought, Hold on a minute. I certainly had strong ideas about teaching and research and what kind of people I'd like to see around me. I was probably as qualified as anyone to build the department. Maybe there was something here that would be worth doing after all. I didn't have to make a decision instantly; maybe I should talk to some people first.

The first one I called was Bob. I told him about my discussion with the dean. "Can you come over to my office?" I said. "It looks like it may be between you and me, and I think we should really talk about it ourselves first."

Bob came over and sat down, but the conversation was strained and didn't last long. I thought it could have been friendlier and more open. Then I called a couple of friends on the faculty to get their opinions and advice. When I went back to see the dean on Monday morning, I still hadn't decided what to do. I thought I'd see how our discussion went, then tell him I needed more time to think it over.

But when I sat down in the dean's office, he didn't ask me if I'd come to a decision or anything else either. He just said, "Joycelyn, I've decided to appoint Bob Fiser chairman." That was it. There was nothing to talk about.

When I left that office, I was seething. I felt totally used. It was obvious to me that the dean's overture on Friday hadn't been real. I was sure that he had asked me for one reason, so he could check off "black" and "female" on the list of those who had been under consideration. That was a deception that had me tasting bile. Plus I had gone and embarrassed myself by talking to people as if I were under legitimate consideration. This thing was giving me some moments of real anger. Given the timing, it seemed a damned good bet that Bob Fiser had been formally offered the position before I asked him in to talk, which would explain why he had acted so strange and uncomfortable. I knew I was going to have to go through some serious changes over this one.

After that, having Bob as my chairman wasn't the most comfortable situation for either of us. I was working on two or three NIH research grants with my own lab people, so while I might not have been the tail wagging the dog, I did have a pretty solid independent base. But Bob and I still had to work through our relationship, which sometimes was a formidable proposition. Through it all we managed to stay friends, though some people might have called us fighting friends. I personally thought of it more like a brother and sister who have a feud going at the moment but who will come to each other's rescue if a true emergency pops up. Which was what happened on a couple of occasions. We'd fight like cats and dogs, but if he got in a real hole or I did, the other one would be there. We also both were very edgy about anyone else talking about the other one. We figured nobody had a right to talk about us except us. The gist of it was that we always managed to work together on essential issues, but most often we kept out of each other's way.

One day early in the summer of 1987 Bob asked me into his office. In the years he had been back in Arkansas Bob had made quite a few political friends, including Hillary and Bill Clinton. I knew that, as did everyone, but I was still surprised when he started telling me that he and Governor Clinton had been reviewing child health issues in Arkansas and that Clinton was intending to reinvigorate the state health department. According to Bob, Clinton wanted to know if I would consider becoming the new health department director.

My first reaction was to wonder if this man thought I had just fallen off the turnip wagon yesterday. If Bob Fiser was promoting me with Clinton, you could rest assured it was not for the betterment of mankind; it was to get me out of the medical school. What also occurred to me was that Bob might have an interest in trying to get control over the health department himself and that he might somehow think my being director there would give him an avenue. After all, a lot of what the health department did was pediatrics: immunizations, child health care, lots of rural obstetrics. If you were politically minded, and you were head of pediatrics at the state medical school, you might think it just made sense for you to be running the rest of the state's pediatrics too.

That was my suspicious side talking. But even leaving Bob out of this, I had never seen the health department on my personal horizon. When I thought of the health department, which wasn't frequently, what I mainly thought of was baby shots and regulating the water supply. They looked after drinking water and septic tanks and restaurant kitchens. Then, if there was an outbreak of salmonella or something, the papers would be shouting, "Oh, the horrible health department," for a day or two. After that you wouldn't hear anything about them until somebody started hitting on them for the next semicrisis that came along.

The health department was not exactly on the cutting edge of medicine. Being director there was not something someone gave up a professorship at the medical school for. The current director was Dr. Ben Salzman, who was in his seventies. Dr. Salzman was a wonderful man, widely liked and admired. He had been a family practitioner who, years and years ago, had joined the medical school faculty and eventually become chairman of the family medicine department. Then, when it came time for him to step down, they had arranged the state health department directorship for him. Was this what I was supposed to be doing at age fifty-four?

While I was thinking all this, I remembered I had actually had a communication with Governor Clinton about the directorship years earlier, right after he had come into office. At that time he had fired the sitting director to make way for someone he wanted to bring in. The man he had fired was Rex Ramsey, a pediatrician I knew and liked, in addition to which I thought he was really doing a good job. It made me blush to remember it, but I had sat down and written Clinton a blistering letter, telling him what I thought he should be looking for in a state health director and why what he had done was so extremely contrary to what he should have done.

One day, a little while after Bob had broached the subject with me, I got a call from a Mr. Tom Butler, who introduced himself as deputy director of the health department. Could I make time for him to come up and see me at the medical school? When Tom came in, we had a nice chat about what the health department was doing and what some of its big challenges were. Tom was articulate and polite. He spoke in a soft drawl and had a muted, businesslike kind of personality. He had been deputy director under several directors and obviously knew everything there was to know. But he didn't exactly do much to arouse my enthusiasm, even though he told me later that the whole point of his coming over was that he was supposed to sell me on taking the job.

My big problem wasn't taking the job. I didn't want the job. But on the other hand, this was the governor asking me to do it. If I were absolutely pushed to the wall on this, I might have to take it, if only as a favor to him; it certainly wouldn't be any favor to me. If that happened, I thought, I'd have to find a way to accept for a short term, then get back to the med school. I didn't like being put in this kind of situation. What would really make sense here would be to find a way to turn him down without actually having to say no.

About a week after Tom Butler visited, Clinton himself called to make the offer officially. He truly hoped, he said, that I was giving serious consideration to what he was asking. I said, "Governor, do you by any chance remember that letter I wrote to you after you fired Dr. Ramsey?"

And he said, "Yes, as a matter of fact I do."

And I said, "Well, I've been thinking about it, and I don't fit a single one of the characteristics that I told you you needed in a health director."

And he said, "I know. But here's why I want you to do it anyway." Then he gave me a little set speech about all the innovative things he wanted the health department to start doing and how he needed someone like me to jump their engine and move them off into new directions. In light of all this, he said, would I take the job?

Having had so much time since Bob Fiser initiated the discussion, I had thought up what I considered a pretty elegant way to get out from under, even though I wasn't comfortable about it since it wasn't exactly straightforward. "The only way I'll consider it," I said, "is if I get to keep my appointment at the university. I also need a ten percent raise in salary. Also, I have to know from you that I would have complete one hundred percent control over the department. If you can get all that, I might do it." Given the precedents involved and the salary figures and the rest, I was pretty sure this was the last I was going to hear from Bill Clinton about the health department.

"Well," he said, "let me see what I can do on those." Then he hung up.

Three weeks or so later the phone rang at about eleven o'clock at night. I was asleep, of course. I had been keeping farm hours for years, and just about anyone who had any business calling me knew that. I never got any calls after nine or so unless there was some emergency. This time it was no emergency; it was Bill Clinton. I *knew* he knew my hours. By now I had served on enough governor's commissions so we had a working acquaintance. "Joycelyn?" he said. "You know all those things you said to get? Well, I got them. So, will you take it?"

I said, "Oh." I said, "I told you I might, didn't I?"

He said, "Yes, you did."

I said, "Oh, well . . . I guess I don't want to lie. . . ."

"Well, that's real good," he said. "Thanks a lot, Joycelyn. Bye, now."

———

One thing about having to become director of the health department: At least Oliver and I didn't need to move anywhere. The department headquarters was about a mile away from my offices at Children's Hospital, right across from War Memorial

Stadium. Tom Butler down there was awfully nice when he started calling me about when I thought I could begin; this was in late July. It sounded like my presence was required yesterday, but I put him off. I told him I'd start October 1.

I used almost all that time closing down my lab and turning my patients over, doing the things I had to do to get out of being a professor for twenty-five years, even though I was only going on leave of absence. Then, on Friday evening, September 28, I took my purse and briefcase, left everything else the way it was, and locked the door to my office on the way out. When Monday morning came, instead of going to Children's, I drove down 630 a little farther, got off at the Pine-Cedar exit, and at eight o'clock sharp walked into the health department building.

My concept of the first day was that I would spend it getting acquainted with everybody. I'd sit down at my new desk, have a cup of coffee, adjust my nameplate, and get people in to talk. After that I'd have a long head-to-head with Tom Butler. Tom had been running this thing for years. I wanted him to fill me in on the current agenda; then, once I had a grasp of that, I could begin thinking about what the longer-range issues were. I knew it was going to take me awhile to get oriented and figure out what needed to be done here and how I was going to do it.

By eight-oh-five I had found my office and was just sitting down when Tom came through the door, not agitated exactly but kind of rushed. "Dr. Elders," he said, "we've got this letter from the governor's office that we've got to get answered by noon. It's about using the Arkansas River for drinking water."

"Yes?" I said. "Tell me about it."

"Well, the river water hasn't been used for drinking or irrigation since the thirties, and now the regulations prohibit it. But they're being questioned. Our water engineers have drafted a response already. If you could just look it over and sign it, that would take care of everything."

As soon as I looked at the letter, I knew I didn't want to sign it. The engineers were giving all the reasons why the river couldn't be used except in times of drought. But I thought, if it could be used during droughts, when the water level was lower and the contaminant level was up, then why couldn't it be used in ordinary times? Besides, I didn't know anything about the background of this. Why did I have to answer it now? Did Tom Butler think I was just going to start rubber-stamping things the minute I walked in the door? "Tom," I said, "I don't understand everything they're saying here, and I'm not sure I agree with it. I'm not signing this like it is."

He stared at me for a moment and blinked. Then he said, "Okay, Dr. Elders, I'd better get everybody up here to explain it to you."

Ten minutes later the office was awash with engineers and chemists spreading out charts and tables and figures all over the place. The basic story was that because the Arkansas River hadn't been used for half a century, some of the counties along its banks were having to transport their water in from long distances. That inhibited their industrial development and population growth. So every year or two they petitioned for a change and brought up a bill in the legislature. The health director then had to advise the governor, which was what I had to do, statutorily, by noon.

For the next almost four hours there was more talk and debate about EPA regulations and bacteria counts and biomonitoring techniques than I had ever heard in my whole previous life put together. The engineers were trying to convince me to sign off, but the problem was that I knew enough chemistry so I didn't convince easily. I pored over the numbers on how much the river had been cleaned up and how it compared with other drinking water sources and argued with a half-dozen experts about conditions under which the river could be used. With all the noise and the crush of data, it wasn't until eleven fifty-five that we reached a compromise and drafted a reply to the governor I could sign. When they all finally cleared out of there, I felt like I needed to cool down.

Instead of that, Tom had me scheduled for lunch with the department's heads of community health programs and maternal/child health. The next thing I knew I was sitting with these people I had never met, looking at the funding we were going to be providing for an array of outside programs: homeless shelters, cooperative health units, the Arkansas AIDS Foundation, and others. A review committee had made the selections, but final approval was up to the director. It was pretty clear by this time that they all had held off on every significant decision until I arrived, and now the water was about ready to burst the dike.

The department heads were briefing me on our list of programs, which all seemed more or less straightforward until we got to an AIDS education grant that was supposed to go to a gay and lesbian organization. "Oh," I heard, "there could be a real bad flare-up over this one, Dr. Elders. We could get some serious criticism here. They've put out a good proposal, and I think they'd do excellent work, but if we fund them, there's going to be political fallout. Of course, it's *your* decision, Dr. Elders." The whole rest of the discussion that phrase kept popping up: It was *my* decision. Try as I might, I wasn't getting any clear advice, except on whose decision it was, which I already knew. The gay and lesbian group had a good track record. On the other hand, the new legislative session where they were going to be debating our budget was coming up soon. Right now might not be the best time to look like we were encouraging homosexuals by giving them money. Then again, it was *my* decision.

"We're going to fund this group," I said. "Whatever the political fallout is, we'll just take it."

"That's excellent," said Debbie Bryant, the maternal/child health chief. "Next is that we're applying for money from the Robert Wood Johnson Foundation to address the infant mortality rate, the maternal death rate, and the teenage pregnancy rate. Now here's the story on that."

By the time I heard the story on that my brain was whirling and I was wondering where in the world I had been for the last twenty-five years. I knew we had a lot of teenage pregnancies in Arkansas, but Debbie was telling me we had the second-highest rate in the country. The same for illegitimate births. And our maternal death rate was more like a third world than a first world country. The same for our infant mortality rate.

While we were talking, I began having flashbacks to my infant wards, especially when I was chief resident and seeing all the new admissions personally. There were times I had twenty to thirty babies with diarrhea and dehydration, all of them hooked up to IVs, with seven or eight more coming in a day. I could still see their sunken eyes and parched skin, with all the subcutaneous water gone. That was dysentery, mostly caused by poor drinking water. Shigella, E. coli, salmonella, amoebic, you name it, we had it. And these were all babies from right around Little Rock; nobody referred dysentery cases from the really poor areas, like the Ozarks or the delta. Then there were our patients with cholera, which you truly associate with somewhere like Bangladesh, and our infants with neonatal tetanus, which you don't ever expect to see outside a textbook. I hadn't known the statistics Debbie Bryant was running through for me, but I had a pretty good visual picture of what they meant.

When I got back from lunch, I asked Tom Butler in and told him some of the things going through my mind. He shook his head a little, with a kind of resigned tolerance, like someone who had gotten tired of being surprised by what other people didn't know. "Dr. Elders," he said, "just as soon as we have a chance, we need to get you around the state and let you see some of the conditions. But first of all, let me tell you about what we've got to do for our budget presentation."

By now I had decided I was going to keep Tom Butler, which I hadn't been sure of before. I knew Tom had a reputation for competence and absolute loyalty, but I also knew he was used to running the show. Six years earlier Dr. Salzman had been brought in as director to calm everybody's nerves and reestablish the health department's relationships after his volatile predecessor had thrown the whole place into an uproar and alienated half the state. While Dr. Salzman was rebuilding bridges, he more or less gave Tom free rein to run the department. If that's what Tom was used to doing, I wasn't sure I was going to be able to work with him. But I liked the way he had handled the river water situation. He hadn't tried to pressure me into signing the letter; he had just swallowed hard, then herded everybody up.

I also liked the remodeling job he had done with his office. When I walked in that morning, my office was right where it had been when I visited the department two months earlier: on the north end of the fifth floor. Tom's, I made a point to notice, was on the south end, just down the hall from me. That was different from where it had been the last time I saw it, which was on the first floor, in the middle of all the traffic and as far away from the director's office as he could physically get it.

I had told Tom then that I was going to have my office down where he was. I was not going to be up in some ivory tower by myself where I had a good view of the outside scenery. "Well," he said, "I don't know what we can do about that. That's where the director's office has always been. Besides, there's no room for you to move down here."

"That's all right," I said. "I'll just take this little office right over here next to your secretary's, where the boxes are."

And he said, "Well, but we can't—you can't have that kind of office."

Tom argued until I said, "Look, you can be wherever you want. But this is what I'm gonna do. The only way I'm ever going upstairs is if you're up there with me." This was in August. Obviously Tom had decided that I meant it because he had moved himself and all the department's business right up to where the action was going to have to flow around me as well as him. That was a pretty good sign we were going to be able to live together, which, as it turned out, was about the best thing that could have happened to me.

"Anyway," Tom was saying, "on the budget presentation. We're already in October. In January the legislature goes into session, and we've got to have everything we want on the agenda. We've been putting the figures together, so I'm ready to go over them with you to whatever extent you might want to." As the department's chief executive Tom had always been the one who presented the budget. He was taken aback when I told him that I would be presenting it this time. Tom's expression didn't change, but I knew he must be wondering when all this was going to end. I had been inside the building only a few hours, and it had just been one thing after another. "Dr. Elders," he said, "you can't present the budget. It's too complicated. They'll be asking all these questions, and you don't know the answers."

"Tom," I said, "then you better start teaching real hard. I'd hate for the health department to lose their whole budget. But if I can't present the budget, I can't be the director. So you-all better get busy. Besides, what do you think these legislators are going to ask me that's more difficult than what those smart young medical students have been asking me all these years?"

That was the start of my nonstop graduate education in how a public health department works and how it's budgeted. Each of the division directors sent me the figures for his division. Then each came in and described for me everything he did, everything he wanted to do, and how much funds were needed for all of it, from long-range objectives down to daily outlays. I said, "If you can convince me on the merits, I'll change my mind about anything. If you can't, I'm not going to do it." At first each division head would give Tom this perplexed look when I said something like that. But before long they all got the idea that they were going to have to argue and fight with me personally about what they wanted. It took a month before I came up for air sufficiently that Tom could start driving me around and letting me see what he called the conditions.

———

Arkansas has seventy-five counties, from Arkansas County to Yell, and each of them has at least one public health clinic while some have two, 106 all told. Over the next four or five weeks I visited every clinic in the state from the Ozarks to the delta, sometimes with Tom, sometimes by myself. By then I was already getting a grasp on what the main problems were. But I wanted to see them for myself, and I wanted to talk to the clinic staffs and home care nurses who were dealing with these things every day.

One of the first offices I went to was Forrest City, Area 9, ninety miles east of Little Rock in the middle of the Mississippi

Delta. I went with Tom, driving down through the black soil flatlands with their soybeans and yellow-topped rice and fields of cotton. This was in the fall, and the harvest was beginning. Huge rice combines were out in the fields, and the automatic cotton pickers that had pretty much replaced the kind of cotton picking I had done as a child and teenager, with my kerchief around my head and the sack trailing over my back. The crops stretched out on either side of Interstate 40 as far as you could see, but there were few people picking them, which was all you really had to know about the economic conditions down there.

When we got to the Forrest City office, I met Louise Dennis, the area manager, and mingled with her people over coffee and doughnuts. Then I gave them my pep talk. Most of these public health workers hadn't seen a department director in years, if they had ever seen one. They were laboring in obscurity, with little recognition for the wonderful work they did every day and no real hope that anything was going to change for the better.

I told them I was pleased to be their new director. I knew there were major problems. I knew they had been out there working far longer than I had and they knew far more about the problems. "I want you to know," I said, "the director's office is open. Anytime you want to call to let me know about something, I want you to do it. I intend to work on the problems with you. We are never again not going to do something necessary because we don't have the money. Never again. You just go out there and get started. You go out there and go as far as you can. And when you can't go any farther because you are out of money, then you call me. It becomes my job then. Until then it's your job to get it done. I am your mouth, but you are the hands and the backbone, and together we're the brain. We've got to improve our immunizations. Thirty-nine percent immunizations is not acceptable. We've got to do whatever we've got to do to get it up to sixty-five percent. You let me know what we can do to help you get that up. You let me know what we can do to get your prenatal people in. You let me know what we can do so you can start trying to reduce your teen-age pregnancy."

They loved it; they stood up and cheered, which charged me up. Clinton had talked about rejuvenating the department. But I got the feeling from Louise's people and from all the others I started visiting that they didn't need rejuvenating. All they needed was for someone to shake things up at the top and give them goals. These people were raring to go.

Louise Dennis, who ran the delta, was a well-bred white woman who came from a wealthy, political family. She had been a public health worker for thirty years plus. Public health was in her bones. Louise had gone out to homes to give children TB medicine or bring them into the clinics for treatment because they didn't even have a horse or mule to come in by themselves. She had given sponge baths to eldery, bedridden sharecroppers and begged milk from storekeepers to feed infants. She had done it all, this very refined, fiftyish, polished white woman with her elegant manners and educated speech, the kind of person you would expect to see at cocktail parties rather than on dirt roads in some backcountry cotton patch. She did go to those cocktail parties—that was her circle—but she was also out in those unpainted shotgun shacks, making sure barefoot children took their medications.

When I got to know Louise better, I understood it was her background that helped make her so good. She and her family had helped elect the local politicians. She knew the mayors and the aldermen and the state representatives and senators. I loved to watch her sitting next to them at some affair and in her finest, most languid drawl with just a touch of lisp say, "Senator Cunningham? We need a few things from you? Which I know you won't mind seein' we get, since we need them so badly?" Louise seemed almost antebellum in her long, stately dresses with the patterns and ruffles and high collars. "Senator Cunningham?" She'd smile. "That's just so very good of you? To do this for us?" Louise Dennis was dynamite on two legs.

Louise drove me down to Marianna first, to visit the clinic there. As I got to see over the next few weeks, many of the public health clinics were located anywhere there was room. They were in unused schoolhouses, storefronts, and every kind

of dilapidated old public building there was. The one in Marianna was in a Civil War–era jail. Louise had been trying to get a new one built for years, with no success. In Marianna, she told me while we were driving, they saw more kids than anywhere else in her area. What they could really use would be a clinic in the elementary school because that's where the children went every day by bus and it was hard for their parents to get them into town on their own. Then she told me about the illegitimacy rate and the STD (sexually transmitted disease) situation and the prenatal care problems. By the time I climbed out of that car after riding half an hour with Mrs. Louise Dennis, I was considerably more educated than when I had climbed in.

Marianna was a typical sunbaked delta town with a big town square and a high pedestal in the middle with Robert E. Lee looking down from it. It was an old-fashioned place where whites owned everything and blacks were field hands—if they could get the work—exactly as it had been seventy-five years ago.

The clinic was in an old stucco building that no one had bothered to tear down after the new courthouse and jail went up, right up the hill. Inside, it had the smell of age and the hundred-year-old heavy oak furniture that always comes with such places. The windows of the jail rooms were barred, and scabrous green paint was peeling off the walls. The nurses had taken burlap and made curtains to cover the bars and dress the place up. Here and there someone had found a reason to put up wallpaper.

Nine or ten nurses worked in this place, and when we walked in, the day was in full swing. In Marianna it was WIC day— women's, infants' and children's food supplements. Poor women had come in with their children to pick up supplies of formula and cartons of baby food. The nurses introduced me around, and I talked to the mothers who were in there, asking them where they were from, how many children they had, how old they were. I knew the health department was providing 65 percent of the formula consumed in Arkansas, which gave you an idea of how many children were being born into poverty. Out in Marianna those statistics had faces you could look at and talk to. Afterward Louise and I sat down to have coffee with some of the nurses in a dark back room with bars and an ominous hook up in the middle of the ceiling. This used to be the hanging room, they told me. Now they gave shots there on immunization days.

Next Louise drove me to Helena on the Mississippi, where it was STD day. Then we went down to Elaine, where the clinic was a storefront crowded with pregnant women waiting for prenatal checkups. Down here in the delta all the patients were black. When I visited up in the Ozarks, it was the same storefront or jail or abandoned public building, but the crowd of pregnant women was white and the men with secondary syphilis or herpes lesions were white. Between the poor whites and blacks there was no difference. Large families, teenage pregnancies, incest, abuse, lack of nutrition, scant medical care. No hopes and no horizons. It was all the same. One was like a photo negative of the other.

———

Sometimes, instead of visiting clinics, I went out with the home health nurses, going to seven or eight houses a day. The thing that impressed me most was how these nurses treated their patients with so much dignity and respect. Many of them had been working their areas for years. They had lived around these poor people for a long time, and they understood them. They had delivered their babies; they had gotten their birth control pills. They didn't just come by once in a blue moon; they knew these families. They knew they had outdoor privies. They knew that they didn't have running water and that there were eighteen of them living in one house.

The home health nurses followed their usual routines, except now they had me in tow. We'd go in someplace, examine a baby, maybe change a catheter or an IV, or give someone cancer medication. Mostly these were ordinary visits. But often out there in the countryside I saw a lot more than I was ready to see.

I remember one day so clearly. We went to visit this thirteen-year-old girl up near Gentry for a six-week postpartum checkup. Before we went in, the nurse told me she suspected the girl was pregnant again. She was living with six men in a very confused situation. Inside, the nurse examined the girl and took a urine sample; then, as we were walking out to the car, a twenty-five- or thirty-year-old man came out of the house, wanting to talk to the nurse too. "You have to do something about her," he said. "She's got something, and we think she's givin' it to all the rest of us too."

Another day I was in a clinic in the Ouachitas watching pre-natal exams and talking with some of the women. There was a young teenager there, and the social worker was pushing to get the name of the father, which the girl did not want to give. I didn't think the social worker was coming on too harshly; it was more gentle persuasion. But finally it just got to be too much for the girl, and she started crying. "It's my grandpa," she said. "He's doing the same thing to my sisters too."

Afterward the social worker told me, "I was pretty sure of that, Dr. Elders. I just thought you needed to hear it too."

Maybe I did or maybe I didn't. When that girl said what she did, I felt hot with shame. I thought about that little Mary, the thyroid case I treated when I was a resident, the one I just let go back home where her father and uncles were "using" her, because I couldn't think what else to do. I don't know that I had thought about Mary for a while. I didn't like to. Whenever I did, it made me cringe. The laws had changed now so you could report such things, but the social worker was having a hard time with this one. There was no father in the house, and the mother knew what the grandfather was doing. "She doesn't think it's a big deal," the social worker told me. "She says he did the same to her. I'd have him arrested, but the problem is he's the only breadwinner. What happens to the rest of them if we go and lock him up?"

Outside Helena I was taken to an unpainted shack sitting out in the middle of a sea of mud, exactly like Schaal in mud season. Inside was a young teenager taking care of what looked like a crowd of babies and toddlers—seven of them when I got a count—when she obviously should have been in school. One of them was hers; the others belonged to her mother and sisters.

The house reminded me of ours, and the girl put me in mind of myself, taking care of our babies, except that I never had more than one or two at a time and Mama would have keeled over dead before allowing me to miss school because of them. But this girl wasn't going to school. She hadn't been since she had her own baby, and she didn't know when she might go back. I knew, though. She was never going back. There was nothing I didn't know about that girl's future.

After one particular day in Governor Clinton's hometown of Hope I was so appalled I couldn't get to sleep at night. My area manager there had arranged for me to talk with a class of boys at the high school, and the questions they asked floored me. "You can't get a girl pregnant, Dr. Elders, if you do it standing up, can you?" Many didn't believe you could. They thought a girl couldn't get pregnant if it was her first time. There was a general impression that if they had an erection with a girl but didn't have sex, something terrible would happen to them. These were boys, many of them already sexually active, who had almost no knowledge of the physiology of sex and no idea about contraception. They understood nothing about protection. I talked about condoms with them. They knew about them. They had heard that they would break, that they would tighten around your penis, and that if you used them too much, they would make it rot off. They had heard that condoms might come off inside a girl and get stuck and that she could die of it.

If I was anywhere within striking distance of Little Rock when I finished my rounds for the day, I'd drive home. Oliver hated me to be driving around late. He was afraid for my safety, much more than I was. But he also tended to get in late himself from coaching. Often we'd go to bed without a word, both of us exhausted. But I wasn't getting much sleep. I was mad, and I was getting madder. I'm probably still mad. Oliver really took the brunt of it. In the middle of the night I'd be grinding my teeth over something and I'd hear, "What's wrong, Sug? You want to talk?"

So I'd start talking: "Oh, Oliver," I'd say, "just listen to what I saw today. . . ."

Among other things, all this had me thinking about the life I had been living the last twenty-five years and what a tiny scratch on the surface I had been making with that. I had just been full of pride about my laboratory and my professorship, but from where I was sitting now the glow didn't look that bright. I used to think that being a professor at the medical school was about the most important thing a person could do in the world. Now I began to see that in the total realm of people's needs what I had been doing hadn't made very much difference at all.

What hit me like a mule kick was how familiar so much of this was. I had been away from conditions like this for a long time. For the last half of my life I had been a doctor living a nice, easy middle-class existence. But I still knew all about it. It was all sitting there in the back of my brain; I just hadn't thought about it. My mind had been somewhere else: on my patients and students, on my research. Maybe I hadn't wanted to think about it. Or maybe I didn't truly understand that people actually lived like that anymore.

But I hadn't forgotten either. Seeing these places was taking me right back to where I had come from. I could identify with all of it. I wasn't looking at these scenes and saying, "Oh, my goodness gracious, isn't this just terrible?" I had lived through it. I didn't have to think, How in God's name do these people survive? I knew how they survived. They survived the same way we had survived. Ignorant and without help. Like my father riding off on the mule with Bernard in his arms. I'd be telling Oliver the things I was seeing, telling him and thinking, There but for the grace of God, Sug, there but for the grace of God.

Chapter 16

The Gordian Knot

I was mad enough so I was talking to myself. And what I was saying was: "I've just got to do something about this. I've got to do everything I can to make people know about it and get involved." I saw these poor, powerless souls, and I thought, They need someone to speak for them; they need a voice. And I mean I was going to push everybody I could find to make people hear me, to make them know, and to make them move.

Here's what I saw. Number one, a whole array of problems from prenatal straight through to the homebound elderly, each problem compounded by ignorance, poverty, and lack of basic services. Number two was all these committed public health people I had: nurses and social workers and doctors who had dedicated their lives to caring for the poor people who needed them. They were a force; they just had to be powered up. Number three, I had 106 public health clinics. Plus we had thousands of schoolhouses where Arkansas's children went every day. Where better to get them screened and treated and immunized and educated about their health—if we could just get ourselves set up to do it?

Meanwhile I was huddled up practically day and night with Tom Butler and my bureau chiefs, working out our budget, which I had to present in January. In Arkansas the legislature

234

is part-time. It meets only once every two years, which meant that whatever budget got passed now was the budget I was going to have to live with until the next session.

In trying to figure all this out, I knew my strength was that while I was no expert on public health, I had been taking care of children for many years, which included paying close attention to their parents and their social and physical environments. So I was used to looking at pathology as something more than just a specific problem of a particular child.

The difference was that before I had always been caring for one case at a time. Now I had problems that couldn't be solved by treating one patient, then the next. I didn't have patients to care for anymore; I had a community, which meant mobilizing the resources of the community. What should the churches be doing? The schools? The businesses? How could I use the media to help me reach my objectives? The problems of maternal care, teenage pregnancy, disease prevention, and the others were interrelated; you couldn't deal with them serially or piecemeal. No one little thing I did was going to make a difference. The question was how to put together this whole pie and get everybody out there focused on it. Because that was what I felt we needed to do if we weren't just going to keep on treading water.

I tried to get myself educated. I spent every spare moment reading, and one book that struck me was Lisbeth B. Schorr's *Within Our Reach*. The reason this book stuck out was that while most experts on public health advocated one strategy or another, Schorr's position is that for poor children, single strategies will not work. Poverty is tied to lack of education, which is tied to lack of contraception, which is tied to teenage and out-of-wedlock births, which are tied to children being raised in poverty, which is tied to lack of education—a great linked chain with little subsidiary links like low-birth-weight babies and congenital malformations and low immunization rates and high sexually transmitted disease rates, and domestic violence and sexual abuse, and two dozen others. Since multiple problems are involved, Schorr says, multiple strategies are required. That got embedded in my brain.

So the question became, What strategies? I put together a conference to look at strategies for dealing with children, to which we invited Schorr and experts from the Carnegie Foundation and Kaiser Institute and others. I also got myself invited to a conference on infant mortality at Amelia Island, Florida, a kind of brainstorming session with some U.S. senators and others concerned with public health. At the same time, of course, I was talking every idea through with Tom and my executive assistant, Jennifer Hui, who was a great listener and facilitator, all of which was helping me sort things out.

I thought what I was doing was just getting educated. Someone with more political experience might have said I was getting radicalized. That was because the more I understood, the clearer it was that while we needed multiple strategies, the best single way to slice the Gordian knot was by cutting the rate of teenage pregnancy. And anybody who looks seriously at teenage pregnancy and what can be done to prevent it becomes a radical in some people's eyes—whether she has any intention to or not. So although I didn't know it, my career as a so-called far-out left radical was about to commence.

In 1987 the United States had the highest rate of teenage pregnancy in the industrialized world, as it still does. As Debbie Bryant had told me my first day at work, Arkansas had the second-highest teenage birth rate in the United States, right next to Mississippi. We knew that 80 percent of children born to unmarried teenagers would be living below the poverty line. That meant each one of those babies increased the welfare costs, increased the health care costs, increased the burden on all the systems necessary to support those children.

Plus, when an unmarried teenager gives birth, you don't lose one person, you lose two, because you lose the mother as well as the child. Teenage pregnancy was the major single cause of poverty and ignorance. Young women who got pregnant lost their opportunity for an education. That meant they were relegating themselves to being slaves, because if you have no education and no money and no hope, that's what you are, a slave. Your life doesn't belong to you; it belongs to the welfare system.

These young girls were cutting off all their opportunity before they even knew what the world was like. Half the time they didn't even know that there was a world beyond where they were. They lived in a town of 200, thirteen miles from a town of 5,000 and they had never been to that big town. Some of them lived fifteen miles from the Mississippi and had never seen the river. The only things they knew were the cotton patch and the backwoods where they were. And if you don't know that there is anything else out there, anybody who comes along looks good. These were young people with no chance, children who have children, who were going to have children themselves, perpetuating that pattern on and on.

To break this cycle, you have got to make a hard investment. And where you have to put your money is in education. Education is prevention. If I can keep them from getting pregnant, I thought, I have a chance to get them educated. And if I can get them educated, they have a chance of making it and living independent, productive lives. But without education their chances went from slim to nil.

I knew that if we could do something dramatic about the problem of teenage pregnancies, we could make a real impact on our state. The question was, How could you get teenagers to stop having babies? Now, the answers to that aren't hard. You have to educate them about sexuality so they have the knowledge necessary to act responsibly, and you have to see to it that if they are going to be sexually active, they know how to protect themselves.

The "how" part didn't take a rocket scientist, but the "where" part was something else. You couldn't educate teenagers at school apparently because some people had the insane idea that if you talked about sex, that was the same as telling them it was all right to go out and have sex. The home might be the ideal place for children to learn about sex and responsibility, but many parents have a hard time talking about sex with their children. So even though maybe it should have been happening in the family, it wasn't, not nearly enough anyway, as the teenage pregnancy figures showed.

It wasn't happening in church either. Far too few churches had sexual education programs for young people. Almost no churches I knew of had really taken on that responsibility, though some of the bigger ones did have a youth pastor who talked to youngsters from time to time. But I did not personally know of a single church that had a good program going on regularly. Besides, 52 percent of Arkansas's children didn't even belong to a church, so how could it possibly happen there?

So no one was educating young people about reproduction and contraception and protection from disease. Not the schools, not the home, not the churches, and certainly not the health department. By the time the girls showed up at the public health clinics, they were already pregnant, which was why they had come. The result was that America's teenage pregnancy rate was more like Mexico's than England's.

Somebody had to start talking about what needed to be done, instead of sitting around wearing a puritanical cloak and wringing her hands. I didn't think this was something where we could afford to mince words either. What I saw was that we were in the middle of a crisis. This need was urgent.

The first thing was to get mobilized. I had Jennifer Hui write up a grant proposal to look at teenage pregnancy. I brought the best people in the business down to Arkansas to talk to us about strategies to deal with teenage pregnancy: Claire Brindis from the University of San Francisco, Kay Johnson from the Robert Wood Johnson Foundation, and Wendy Baldwin from the NIH. We spent three days in a room with them, going through every aspect of our problem. On their recommendation, we organized a statewide conference to focus attention, inviting different people who were worrying about maternal/child health: public health people, teachers, social workers, legislators, ministers. One legislator actually told me, "Dr. Elders, before you started talking about it, we didn't have any teenage pregnancy problem in Arkansas."

By the time we were well into this I knew there were two directions I wanted to go in, and I put them out on the table. One was comprehensive health education, including education about sexuality. As it was, Arkansas had laws on the books requiring health education throughout the school years. But the schools weren't doing it. The law was there, but the schools didn't have the money for it. Instead they'd teach health one semester, usually in eighth or ninth grade.

I wanted the K–12 health education requirement implemented. I wanted students to learn about good nutrition and the dangers of smoking and alcohol and drugs and what it meant to be growing up. I wanted them to know about human reproduction. I wanted the younger ones to know there were places on their bodies that no one should be touching, and I wanted the older ones to be educated about pregnancy and contraception. I wanted these things taught in a regular, age-appropriate way, with the messages reinforced over years so they got ingrained, so that when they got to be teenagers, they would have the background to make responsible decisions.

Everybody knows you don't just say no. That's never the way it works. You have to have the knowledge and the background to be able to say no and to understand why it's important to say no. And if you are going to be sexually active, you'd better understand how to protect yourself against AIDS and other STDs and how to keep yourself from getting pregnant.

All this was just so normal and necessary that it didn't occur to me as a serious proposition that anyone except a fringe group was going to object. We were having an epidemic of sexually transmitted diseases and teenage pregnancy. Would any parents who cared for their children object to teaching them how to protect themselves? On the contrary, there was nothing they wouldn't do to protect their own child from an unplanned pregnancy or AIDS or some other sexually transmitted disease. As I began telling high school kids, "Your parents do not want you having sex. They don't want that. But I'm telling you, they would get up at midnight to go out and buy you a condom themselves if it was a choice between that and you getting pregnant or contracting a disease."

Comprehensive health education K–12 was one direction. The superintendents and principals and PTAs could use existing

239

curricula, some of which, like Berkeley's "Growing Healthy," were very good, or they could pick and choose and figure out locally what they wanted or didn't want. What was important was that they did it. If they didn't have money to hire teachers, I would start raising it for them. I'd go to the budgeting process. I'd look for grants. I would get it somehow.

The second thing I decided to go after was school-based clinics. School-based clinics are medical facilities located in schools that can be used by students and teachers. In rural areas transportation to public health clinics or doctors is often impossible, and in poor areas of both the country and city, few doctors are available. But schools are there already, and so are school buses. Putting medical facilities in schools, staffed by public health people, is the most efficient, least expensive way to get health care to children, period.

I didn't invent school-based clinics. When I started talking about them, the idea was already at least a quarter century old. The first school-based clinic had been funded by the federal government twenty-five years earlier in Minneapolis and was still going strong. Then the Robert Wood Johnson Foundation had given money for pilot programs in various states, and by 1987 there were probably thirty of them up and running in one place or another.

The follow-up studies had proved their success in screening for disease and providing primary treatment. But they had also become controversial. Since clinics located in high schools treated teenagers, a truly bizarre undercurrent of opposition began to form around the idea that these facilities were some kind of subversive attempt to place sex and abortion clinics right inside the schools. This notion was about as rational as the fear back in the fifties that fluoridating water was an international Communist plot. School-based clinics had never done abortions, and in most places the categories of services they provided as well as who could use them were determined locally by parents and school boards.

I knew about the controversy. I wanted our clinics to be able to provide pregnancy counseling and condoms. But even without that, we had a pressing need for primary, preventive health care for our young people. As far as I was concerned, the health department would see that funding was available; I was going to put that in my budget and fight for it. After that the local school boards and parents would make the decisions about who got what kind of treatment, which was the way it was going to be in Arkansas in any case. We had twelve hundred school districts, and each one was autonomous. They were going to decide for themselves whether to have a clinic or not or to provide condoms or not. My job was to do everything I could to publicize the issue and give them the ability to make a decision.

One day after I started going around to see the conditions in the state, Tom Butler told me, "Dr. Elders, at least we don't have to teach you how to be poor." Tom meant that as a compliment. Before I actually showed up, he may have thought I was going to be some kind of distant academic type. There was never much chance of that. But as I began to understand the teenage pregnancy problem, I realized that in a way this really was *my* issue. Most of the adolescents who got pregnant were poor, and the black rate was twice that of whites. Who else could talk to these girls about sexuality like I could? I'm the right color, I thought. I'm the right sex. I've been as poor as poor. "Heavens," I caught myself saying to one group I was addressing, "the only person in the world who can say this or do this is an educated black female. Black men can't do it. White women can't do it. White males sure can't do it. I've got all the tools necessary to take this on. This must be God's mission for me."

While I was gearing up for the budget fight, the governors' association was getting ready to hold a national conference on "Youth at Risk" in Washington, D.C. As part of this effort many of the states were holding their own conferences, including Arkansas, where youth issues were very close to Governor Clinton's heart. I participated, along with many of the other heads of state departments, and afterward there was a big press conference at the Capitol Building. Governor Clinton was standing in the middle with all the various directors lined up around him taking turns talking about what their agencies were going to do for the youth of Arkansas.

The governor had a big investment in education and youth programs, but this particular get-together wasn't on fire with excitement. There were just too many people, sixteen or seventeen directors, reeling off what they had in mind to do, one after the other. By the time it got to my turn most of the room looked like it was dozing off. Then somebody asked me what the health department was going to do for youth, and I said, "We're going to reduce teen pregnancy."

When they heard that, some of the reporters perked up. "Dr. Elders," one asked, "how are you going to do that?"

"Well," I said, "we're going to have comprehensive health education and school-based clinics."

Now they were all wide-awake. Somebody said, "School-based clinics? Does that mean you're going to distribute condoms in schools?"

I said, "Yes, it does. We aren't going to put them on their lunch trays. But yes, we intend to distribute condoms."

The instant I said that they all stopped staring at me and swung their heads over to stare at the governor. So did I. From where I was standing, it looked like his face had turned the color of the sweater I was wearing, which was bright red.

"Governor?" They all were trying to go at once. "Governor, Dr. Elders just said she was going to give out condoms in schools. Do you agree with that? Is that the policy of your administration? Governor?" I knew I had just dropped my governor in an ocean of Jell-O. I was watching him, every bit as interested as the reporters to see what he was going to say.

Governor Clinton looked like he was trying to swallow something. Then after a moment he said, "Well, Dr. Elders told me what she was about before I appointed her. And I support Dr. Elders."

I had several feelings when I heard that. One was satisfaction that he had the courage to support me and not hedge. There was also some humor in it, for me anyway, because while Bill

Clinton and I had enjoyed a good working relationship, we didn't exactly have a thorough review of issues and policies when he asked me to be health director. It was just "Thanks, Joycelyn. Bye, now," at eleven o'clock at night. He didn't have any more idea than I did that I was going to make teenage contraception an issue. But you know, after that Clinton never did budge from supporting me, at least not while we were in Arkansas. Lastly, I appreciated his ability to think on his feet and talk his way out of a hard place. When he was running for President, I used to tell people, "With Bill Clinton you're dealing with a man who knows how to swim in Jell-O."

That was an important press conference for me. In some ways it set the tone for the rest of my public career. Almost right off the people of Arkansas started hearing from conservative religious groups that if I wasn't stopped, their sons and daughters were going to be served condoms on their school lunch trays right along with their lunches.

Bill Clinton might have supported me, but when I got home that night, I wasn't so sure about Oliver Elders. Oliver had heard about the conference on the evening news, along with everyone else in Arkansas. "Aw, Sug," he said when I came through the door. He looked pained. "How could you go and say something like that? You're going to get us run all the way out of town."

The day after that press conference the health department phones started ringing, and they never stopped. Mail began to pour in by the sackful. This was 1987. I never in my life expected that contraception would be such a hot-button issue. I thought there would probably be some argument about distributing condoms. But we were only going to do it for teenagers who had their parents' permission to use the school clinics' pregnancy counseling services. What kind of war did that have to start? But if naïveté can be measured in sackfuls of mail being emptied across your desk, my naïveté level must have been pretty high.

Reading those letters, I found out for the first time in my life that I was an atheist—or, at least, so I was being told. Many of the writers also believed I had no morals or that I was in favor of homosexuality. Others accused me of wanting to teach their little children how to perform sex acts. Some said I was a baby killer. I had always had a good thick hide, but that shocked me a little. At that point I had never so much as mentioned the word "abortion." I was a pediatrician. I had never done one or even seen one. But some people just knew I had to be a baby killer. The mention of condoms and sex education was like a trip wire that set all the abortion sirens going off full blast.

The really ugly letters my secretary, Willie Mitchum, never let me see. She'd say, "Oh, Dr. Elders, that was too bad for you to look at." I wondered what those had in them. The ones Willie was giving me were bad enough. Years later she told my secretaries at the surgeon general's office not to show me the worst. "Dr. Elders gets mad," she said.

At first I was going to try to answer every letter. But it got to be ridiculous, especially when we saw that the vast majority of them were orchestrated. Fifty or a hundred identical letters would come in on the same day, all with the same return zip code. On one occasion they all misspelled the same word. It wasn't hard to figure out this was a letter that had been passed out at church and everyone in the congregation had copied it.

After a week or two of this I decided the way to deal with it was to invite the most vocal callers and letter writers to come in so I could talk to them face-to-face. Most of what I was reading just had no relation to what I truly had in mind to do. I expected that I differed with most of these people. I knew they were opposed to sex education. But I felt they didn't really understand what I was talking about, and I wanted them to understand. I thought that if I had a chance to explain things, I could get them to see the magnitude of the problems we had to deal with. So I invited the Christian Coalition, the Right to Life, Focus on the Family, and the other groups that had written to me to come in for a meeting. Twenty-three invitations in all to the leaders and the most vehement preachers.

The invitation was for December 10 at one o'clock. I reserved the conference room and got myself ready for what I thought was going to be a spirited dialogue. I intended to make converts. If I couldn't do that, at least I wanted to make clear to them the dimensions of our teenage pregnancy problem and what its consequences were. I didn't want their opposition, I wanted to work out some kind of satisfactory solution.

A little after noon on the day of the meeting Tom Butler stepped into my office, nervous. "Dr. Elders," he said, "we've got a lot of folks downstairs who say they've come for the meeting. They're getting to be a whole crowd already. We're never going to get them all into the conference room."

Just then Willie came in on the intercom to say there was a call from Channel 4. Somebody had told the TV people that the health department was holding a public meeting on sex education and condoms. They wanted to know why hadn't we made an announcement. They were sending a crew right down to cover it, and they wanted to set up inside the building. Would it be all right with us if they did that?

I told Willie to tell Channel 4 I'd get back to them. Then I asked Tom to go take another look at what was happening downstairs. When he came back, he said it looked like there was some kind of demonstration going on. Lots of people were milling around out in front of the building and wandering through the downstairs hallways. "Do you want to just cancel it?" he said. "Or we could let the people we invited come up here to the boardroom and see if we can't get the rest of them at least to go outside."

I heard what Tom was saying, but I really wasn't paying much attention. Here I had invited a group of twenty-three leaders and pastors in to have a discussion, and instead they had rigged up a demonstration for themselves, complete with the TV. My first reaction was that it was kind of funny they had done this. My second was just to get them all inside. If they wanted to duke it out, I was ready for that. It didn't occur to me for a moment to call it off. I had never been involved in anything like this before in my life, so I didn't have any preparation for how to handle it. But I for sure didn't feel intimidated, which was probably what they wanted me to feel. "What's going on in the auditorium?" I asked Tom. "If no one's using it, why don't we just move them in down there? Will they all fit?"

I could tell Tom was concerned I might do something crazy like this on the spur of the moment. "Dr. Elders," he said, "you sure you really want to do that?" He thought it might turn dangerous. Also, he had just heard that some state senators, our opponents in the legislature, had shown up. They had been informed too, right along with the media.

I didn't care. Maybe I didn't know enough to care. "Yes, I do," I told Tom. "Just let them all in—but only if they'll sign their names, addresses, and phone numbers. If they want to come in and fight, let them own up to who they are." Then I told Willie to get back to Channel 4 and tell the TV crew they were welcome to set up inside.

Tom left to do what he had to to get the crowd into the auditorium and also to take a few countermeasures of his own, which I found out about a little later. I waited awhile; then I went down. When I got there, the room was packed. I noticed that ten or twelve men from the department were there too, courtesy of Tom, no doubt. There was a lot of noise, but it didn't strike me as a violent crowd. I had the sense that they had come armed with their arguments, and they were planning to convince me I was wrong. Well, that was all right. I was planning to convince them.

I walked down the aisle to the front and went to the podium. The first thing I did was welcome them and thank them for coming. "I want to thank you all for coming down to the health department today. I think it's good you came down here to express your different points of view. We're all intelligent people here who can have an honest and open discussion with each other. I am absolutely sure that all of us in this room want only one thing, and that's to do what's best for our children." Then I talked for five or ten minutes, telling them how I saw the problems and what I intended to do about them.

When I finished, the comments started coming from the audience. First some spokespeople who had obviously come prepared with speeches talked. The first was a woman doctor who had been involved with antiabortion groups for a long time. Then a couple of others. Each of them gave a short dissertation, at the end of which there'd be an uproar of approval from the crowd. Then I answered, giving them my position on it and why what they were advocating wasn't going to do a thing except let the same problems we already had get worse.

After this little group of speakers, the auditorium began to get rowdier and more hostile. Some people had worked themselves up into a real rage. One woman shook her finger at me and declared that sex education was pornography. She had two five- or six-year-old girls sitting next to her. She didn't want anybody teaching her children about "fisting," she said, and something else. I leaned over and said, "Tom, what's fisting?" He told me, but he didn't know what the other thing was she had mentioned. He said he'd have to ask one of our STD people.

While this lady was talking, I noticed my brother Chester sitting there in his Methodist collar. Tom was always wanting to make sure I was protected. I knew he must have called Chester. Lee Lee Doyle was there too, a close friend of mine from the medical school who was a specialist in reproductive physiology. Then Reverend William Robinson walked in. Reverend Robinson was a minister in Little Rock whose church was the meeting place for the Ministerial Alliance, the umbrella group of black churches. He was widely known for his day-care and outreach programs and later was in charge of my minority AIDS program, which served as a countrywide model. Tom had gotten him down there too.

Reverend Robinson and Chester weren't the only ministers in the place. One man with a collar got up and started preaching that God was going to strike me down for teaching children how to have sex. He was calling down hellfire and brimstone. Then he said that there wasn't anybody else who was going to teach his daughter how to have sex, that only he was going to teach her that. It took me a moment before I realized that he was one of this cult we have in Arkansas that believes that adult members of the church have to be the ones to initiate their children. I knew about them. One of my lab technicians had grown up in that cult. Her parents had been part of it, and she had been in therapy a long time trying to deal with it.

The marathon went on for three hours, and when I was getting ready to close it down, one man got up and said, "I feel we need to close with a prayer."

I said, "Sir, this is *my* meeting, and *I* decide how it's closed. Thank you." And that was it.

Afterward the two senators who had been there talked to Tom. One of them was a man from Carlisle whose wife lived in their house while he lived in a trailer in the backyard with his girlfriend. I didn't know what business he had taking a moral position on something. The other was Knox Nelson, who was probably the most powerful politician in Arkansas at the time, more influential than the governor. "Tell the doctor this is too hot," they told Tom. "She needs to just leave it alone."

"You know, Dr. Elders"—this was Tom talking—"these people can destroy our whole budget. There's no percentage in antagonizing them if we can do what we want some other way."

But I was mad. "Tom," I said, "I'm the health director. I'm going to do what I think needs to be done. If that means we might antagonize somebody, we'll just have to take that risk."

The right-to-life groups that had put this show on tried their best to capitalize on it, claiming that the health department had called a public meeting and that those opposed to sex education and school clinics had outnumbered those in favor ten to one. But the meeting had been so wild that they took a beating in the media. The real made-for-television drama wasn't their prepared speakers delivering speeches in opposition; it was the crazies shaking their fingers in my face and spouting about hell and damnation and how sex education was pornography. The result was that for the next month the TV stations showed the worst of them and the best of me. I didn't always have a lot to thank the media for, but I could never really get mad at them either. After that meeting I knew how it worked.

One result of all the coverage was a swell of support for what we were trying to do. More than anything else could, that meeting made people think about who these wild fringe groups were and what they wanted. All over the state the message we were getting was that people did not want to associate themselves with what they were seeing on their TV screens.

But I also realized after that meeting that I probably had more opposition than I had thought. I had run into a pretty good buzz saw. I just had not been aware that all of this very well organized crew was out there. On the other hand, I figured there was a good sampling of them in that room. I felt that most people in the state really agreed with me, not them. And I began to think how I could begin getting people lined up on my side. That's when I decided to go out and start working with the Religious Forum, which was the umbrella group of white churches, and the Ministerial Alliance, the black group. I was ready to fight tooth and nail.

One thing I have to say about all this. I was in a unique position, and it was probably that position that made me so ready to do what I thought needed doing. I was the health director. That was a political appointment and should have been subject to all the usual political pressures. But I was also still a tenured professor at the university, which was one of the requirements I had given the governor. I was just on temporary leave of absence. If all of a sudden Bill Clinton said that he didn't need my services or that these things weren't what he wanted, all I needed to do was say, "Thank you, Governor. Here's my resignation," and go back over to my other job, which I loved and was having a good time at when I left, despite my intramural feuding with Bob Fiser. If I had been in the position of having to worry about getting fired, I might not have taken things so aggressively. But I wasn't in that position, so I didn't worry about it.

———

When Chester took over at Hunter United Methodist, Oliver and I switched from Liberty Baptist. Chester and his wife, Valerie, used to come over every Sunday after services for dinner, and often they'd bring friends along. Then we began having a lot of dinners at the church. I was starting to feel like I was cooking myself to death, so after the first year or so I had to take a rest. But not from actual churchgoing. With Chester in the pulpit it was hard for me to leave my pew empty. Over time I found I was more active in church affairs than I had been for many years.

When I recognized how important it was to take my message to the churches, Chester was the key person. Without an audience you are sure not to make a difference. He got me my audience. Chester's superior, Bishop Wilke, was very supportive. Methodists had always been on the right side on contraception, and he wrote letters to all his district superintendents and ministers. Chester also set me up with the black Ministerial Alliance and the white Religious Forum groups of churches.

My meeting with the black ministers struck some sparks. I stood up in front and told them we had a crisis in our community, and a crisis requires crisis intervention. "I need for you to stand up in your pulpits on Sunday," I said, "and tell your congregations that we need sexuality education, that we need school-based clinics."

One minister got up and said, "That contradicts what we preach. We preach abstinence. We say abstain. Don't do it."

"You've been preaching abstinence ever since you've been preaching," I told them. "At least I believe you have. I know my brother preaches that. But I've still got a problem in Arkansas. I've got eight thousand plus teenagers having babies!"

They talked about the morality of distributing condoms. I told them that it was morally wrong for children to be hungry, morally wrong for children to be cold, morally wrong for children to be abused and that we needed to do something about it.

I took the same message to the white ministers. I thought that as a group they were undecided and sitting on the fence until a Catholic priest got up and said, "You-all know that Dr. Elders disagrees with some of the basic principles of our church. But she's right that we have a crisis in our community that requires crisis intervention. So I support what Dr. Elders is trying to do."

That moved me and most of the others in the meeting. After that they voted to support my efforts.

I didn't know exactly what it meant, that they were going to support me. It might have just meant that they weren't going to oppose me from the pulpit. But a couple of months later when the legislative session opened up, a lot of those men put their collars on and came up to the State Capitol to shake hands with their legislators and twist arms. Black ministers and white. From what I could see, probably more whites than blacks.

By this time it seemed like I was stirring up controversy every time I moved. While I was working to persuade our ministers, I was invited to speak to a gay and lesbian group called One in Ten that was holding a seminar at the medical school. I thought I should. AIDS was a growing epidemic, especially among homosexuals. But gay people were subject to a lot of other problems: ostracism; discrimination; increased depression and suicide rates among teens. Homosexuality was another area I had never given a lot of considered thought to, but these were real problems, and I felt I should speak out about them as I saw them. I thought that was appropriate for the director of public health.

I wasn't the only speaker at the One in Ten seminar. The woman responsible for AIDS education in the department of education was there, and various other people. I spoke about the importance of making school counselors sensitive to the special problems of gay teenagers and the need to educate the community generally that people with a different sexual orientation should be tolerated and accepted. We had to find a way to get over our homophobia.

I know I never heard a word about homosexuality when I was growing up. I never heard a word about any kind of sexuality. But in Schaal we learned a very simple but profound lesson of faith, not just from Mama but from our little Tabernacle Methodist Church. We were taught that above everything we were all equally God's children. "Judge not," the Gospel says, "lest ye be judged." And the reason you didn't, we were taught, was that you never knew what kinds of shoes your neighbor has had to walk in.

So I gave my speech, and the education department AIDS coordinator gave hers. It was the last speech she ever gave in that job. She was eaten alive by the press and the fundamentalists. The department of education, they said, had no right to condone homosexuality, which was their interpretation of her being there. She had no right to speak to this group, and she should be fired, which she was. In my mind I was just daring anybody to say that I didn't have a right to speak. Nobody did. On the other hand, my mail volume started setting new records, just as the legislature was getting ready to convene and begin scrutinizing our budget.

Chapter 17

With Children It's Forever

❦

"We were fixing to go into session in January...." This is Tom Butler speaking now. In the couple of months I had been on board Tom had practically become my alter ego. There were some things we didn't see eye to eye on, but from the very beginning we communicated. We could sit and argue about something till we were blue in the face, but when we walked out of that room, we walked out together. Whatever decision we had reached was the decision, and whether Tom won the fight or not, he put his whole heart into seeing that it got done. The health department was Tom's child. He wanted it to grow and bloom. The last thing in the world he wanted was any sign of internal divisiveness. He was worried enough without any of that.

Tom: "We were fixing to go into session in January, and I was saying to myself, 'Another six months and this director won't be around.' I could see where she was going. She said, 'We're going to do this!' I thought, You couldn't sell that on a bet. I advised her. I said, 'This is good, I'm not saying we shouldn't do it, but we haven't prepared. What you're wanting to do would take a year of selling.' But giving advice to her wasn't like giving advice to other directors. She didn't do things that way. She was a street fighter."

The first senator Tom took me to see was Max Howell, who ruled the roost up at the Capitol. Some politicians have seniority but no power. Max Howell had both. "He'll probably want us to come in there real early," said Tom. "Then he won't see us for a while. But you need to be there because he has this thing about time. Just don't get upset; he does that to everybody." I must admit I was a little bit shaky. Howell had a reputation for being disputatious and overbearing, which didn't bode that well for our getting along. But I knew I needed him. I just thought I better be superprepared to convince him on what I wanted to do for the health department.

Tom again: "Max Howell was the senior legislator, in fact the most senior state legislator in the United States at that point, an old-time country lawyer, gruff, combative, and domineering. I had watched him take people apart for a long time. He and one or two of his cronies would be pulling this way and that till people would start separating at the seams. I expected a real cat-and-dog fight. But he just took to Dr. Elders. It was as if he recognized a fellow spirit. The same with Nick Wilson, one of the up-and-coming powers in the Senate who was also a powerful, authoritarian personality. But he and Dr. Elders also hit it off right from the start."

The thing was that Senator Howell did not like weak people. He'd bite and carry on, as we learned later. When he started asking you questions, if he sensed you were backing down or weaseling, he would slice your head right off. But if you fought back and stood up and defended yourself, he'd say something like "Well, you got your stuff with you today, don't you, Doctor?" He really seemed to like that. He'd turn to his colleagues and say, "Just don't you talk any more to this woman, and don't let her talk. Don't ever let her tell you anything. If she ever starts telling you something, you'll give her the whole damned state."

Senator Nick Wilson was another. He was a lawyer from up at Pocahontas in northern Arkansas. He nipped and griped and just really liked to plaster people against the wall. But he took me under his wing. He would tell me, "Well, I'll try to get that done for you, Doctor." Or, "Why don't we not do this right now?" He wasn't going to take on battles he knew he was going to lose. "Doctor, why don't we just put that back on the stove and let it simmer a little while longer?"

If Nick Wilson or Max Howell told me to go ahead on something or asked me not to do it, I knew I could rely on his judgment. With those two I didn't say, "Well, I'm going to do this anyway," and walk out the door and there it is. We might not necessarily agree on particular issues, but I knew they were going to be straight with me, and they knew I was straight with them.

———

When we finally had the 1988 budget ready to go, it made a book two and a half inches thick. I first presented it in private to Governor Clinton; of course I had kept him apprised of the controversial items like school-based clinics and money for condoms as we went along. Then we took it to the budget committee, which had to approve it before reporting it out to the full legislature. "The committee's only going to let you talk for thirty or thirty-five minutes," Tom told me, so I abstracted all the major points and made slides.

"You can't show slides," he said. "They won't let you do it."

"Well," I said, "why don't you call and ask them?"

When the answer came back yes, I put all the different areas of the state on slides, so the committee members could look up there, see their districts, and then see the problems in their districts: teenage pregnancy, environmental health, the immunization rate, the condition of the health department facilities. We had people go out and take pictures of the health clinics, like the jail in Marianna, by district, so the legislators could see where their own constituents were being treated and look kindly on our request for new clinics.

Tom was so anxious about this slide business that he made me present it to the Arkansas Board of Health first. The board members thought it was so good they all wanted to borrow the slides for their own presentations. But Tom was still anxious. "You don't know how they might act," he said. "Some of them up there can be like little boys at times."

The budget committee had forty or fifty members. Usually they never listen; they like to wander around and talk. When I started out, they got all giggly; they thought this was very humorous. When I turned down the lights, one voice said, "We gonna get popcorn too, Doc?"

"You just sit down there," I said. "If you're good, you'll get some at the end."

While I was taking them through the budget, though, they were quiet. I could tell the visual representations were having an effect. When I was finished, one of them got up and said, "I've been in this legislature thirty-two years, and that's the best budget presentation we've ever had. I recommend we approve the health department budget."

And somebody else said, "Second the motion."

Next thing I knew it was over and Tom was hustling me out of there before I could say something else. That wasn't the last time he did that. At one point in the next session, when I already had some experience, we were fighting in committee for additional in-home health services. But there was an obstinate group opposing us. When Knox Nelson, the chairman, saw how it was going, he tabled the item and told Tom and me to come back next week. Knox often didn't support what we wanted, but sometimes he did, and this was one of those times.

Next week we were there first thing, and Knox said, "Meeting come to order." They were all kind of milling around in back, gossiping and stoking themselves up for round two. "Dr. Elders? You want those in-home health services?"

"Yes, sir," I said, "I do."

Senator Jay Bradford, who was a great advocate of health care, was sitting next to him. "I recommend 'do pass,'" Jay said. "The in-home budget, recommend 'do pass.'"

The legislators at the back were looking up now and starting to move toward their seats.

"Motion pass," said Nelson. "Thank you, Dr. Elders."

"Yes, sir," I said. I was geared up to testify. "I believe—"

But Tom was pulling on my sleeve, whispering. "Let's get out of here. It's over; it's done; you got it. Now grab your bag quick and let's get to the car." After that I figured as long as I had someone like Jay Bradford on my side and Tom to tell me when to get out, I'd bat a thousand.

Tom was a great administrator and manager. He didn't enjoy combat and confrontation, though. So we were good complements for each other. I could stand up and talk and be in the public eye, and he could work his magic behind the scenes and get all the things we wanted. I say *we* wanted, because in retrospect probably about half of what I was out there thinking was mine was really due to Tom's having convinced me. I know, for example, that all of our renovated and new buildings— twenty-eight new public health clinics that we built before it was over—were Tom's idea initially. Tom was not an M.D., which meant that by law he could never be director. But he knew what he was after, and I think he saw me as someone who could help him achieve his goals. Having Tom behind the scenes allowed me to do the visionary and missionary part, and having me out front allowed him to do the manipulating and jockeying part. I think we each thought we had the best of both worlds.

Even so, I know that my style was often a trial to him. I didn't go to the legislature begging. I went in with "You haven't done your job. This is what you need to do. And if you don't do it, I'm going to go out and tell *your* constituents that *you* voted against *their* children!" I did not go out with my hat in my hand, which was how legislators expected department heads to act. I thought they had to be told what was right and then pushed in the direction they needed to go in.

Here's how Tom saw it, which I'm sure goes for my other top advisers too, like Nancy Kirsch and Jennifer Hui. "She would stand right up and say, 'Hey, you're wrong. This is right and you're wrong!' Sometimes there was nothing for us to do but get on and hold tight. She'd start talking in that singsong, and there was no stopping her. She'd just be rockin' and rollin';

she'd take on all comers. Sometimes when we listened to her speak, we'd be sweating bullets."

The real truth is that while I did have some blowups, I didn't have to be real combative in the legislature all that often. The reason I didn't was that the legislators just had no idea how to handle an educated black woman. I understood that early on, and I used it to the hilt. The trick was always to go in super well prepared and to establish a reputation for that. Because the last thing on earth any politician wants is being made to look bad in front of his peers and most especially by a black female. If you get beaten up by another white male, well, that's not good, but it's not terrible. If a white female gets the better of you, that is terrible, but it's not mortifying. But if it's a black female, that's the worst kind of sin imaginable. So even when they disagreed with me, they tended not to be too harsh about it. The idea of being embarrassed by someone like me wasn't really tolerable, so that lent a kind of civility to my debates up there, usually.

Actually, the fact was that while many of Arkansas's legislators used colorful language and liked a good fight, at heart most were gentlemen. I might have had one or two dyed-in-the-wool enemies, but by and large I was able to work with them, right across the ideological spectrum. The press sometime portrayed me as someone unable to compromise. But I don't think there's a legislator in Arkansas who didn't feel we accomplished a lot when I was health director. And what I got, I got through negotiation and giving some to get some, the way you always have to. I might have had a reputation for confrontation, but that was not the basic nature of my relationship with the legislature. That came mostly from my encounters with the extreme groups of the so-called Christian right.

I'm not sure that when I went up as surgeon general, I found Washington very different from Arkansas. I really thought that most of the politicians who were there had a lot of respect, not perhaps necessarily for me, but for the surgeon general's office. The big difference was that I was health director six years and surgeon general only fifteen months. If I had left at the end of fifteen months in Arkansas, I don't know what my final reputation there might have been. I think that if I had had a chance to work with Congress over a longer period of time, I would have gotten along fine with them too. It would have become a productive relationship. Even during my confirmation hearings, many of the Republican senators got up on the floor and said in one way or another, "You've heard this woman is bullheaded and aggressive, but I've never met a more respectful public servant." Which is the way I tend to be personally. "Yes, sir" and "Yes, ma'am" are the vocabulary I was brought up with. It's hard for me to act some other way.

But though that's true, it's also true that the demonstration those right-to-lifers staged in the health department auditorium and the letters I was getting showed me an enemy I had nothing but contempt for. When I invited those people in originally, it was because I had wanted to talk. I was new to all this, and I wanted to sit down together and see what grounds we might have to move issues ahead. That's what I was planning to get out of it. What I did get out of it was that there is a segment of people for whom any discussion of sex education or contraception sets off a tornado of irrationality. For them it all leads straight to abortion. And their discussion of abortion is full of the kind of sanctimoniousness and moral self-righteousness that makes most religious people cringe. What they mainly have is a deep-down need to control other people's lives.

For as long as I have had an opinion on the subject, I have believed in a woman's right to choose. I think reproductive choice is essential. If you can't control your own reproductive life, you can't control your life. So I support choice. I feel it is a decision that is best left to a woman, her significant other, her doctor, and her God. I don't know of anyone else who is good enough, knows enough, or loves enough to make that decision for her. That has always been pretty much all I have ever had to say about it. Our opponents on school-based clinics had decided that I was in favor of having everybody go out and get abortions. But that had nothing to do with what I wanted. I wanted to prevent unplanned, unwanted pregnancies. As I started saying in some of my speeches, I never knew a woman who wasn't pregnant to need an abortion.

I understood that there were serious, intelligent people involved in the antiabortion movement whose faith and integrity I respected, even though I didn't agree with them. But in Arkansas the part of the movement that draws the publicity and gets the exposure is not that sort. The part of the movement you see most down here, that I was seeing all the time now that I was health director, was the ones who hide behind God in order to suppress the ability of poor people to protect themselves from deepening their own poverty and desperation. These were people who never in their lives cared one whit about the welfare of poor people, who never voted for education or medical care or food supplements for families that couldn't feed themselves. Un-Christian people who by some twisted logic believed they should be called Christians. People unaware of the difference between being religious and being Christian. "Very religious non-Christians" I started calling them.

I hadn't run into these people much during my medical school career, but I knew them well enough. They were the same people who in former days were against civil rights and who believed that religion justified segregation and inequality. The worst of them were people who in earlier times wore sheets over their heads, and we called them the Ku Klux Klan. They have been fighting forever, and I recognized them, the same as everyone in the South does whose memory goes back at all. Their fight's not even really about abortion. Does anyone actually think they care if poor black girls have abortions or not? It's not about religion. It's about controlling somebody else's life. They haven't changed; it's just that their old rallying cries aren't fashionable anymore. So they've changed what they're about. But they're the same folk.

January 22 was the anniversary of *Roe* v. *Wade,* and Planned Parenthood was going to be holding a rally in the rotunda of the State Capitol. I was invited to speak there, and I decided to do it. I had no illusions about whom I was fighting and no hesitation. That day I gave as strong a speech as I knew how.

It turned out to be the first of a series of speeches I gave on the anniversary. They all had basically the same theme, but none of them raised more contention than the one I gave in 1992, the year before I was nominated for surgeon general.

A little bit before that one of the extreme fundamentalist churches—the Fellowship Bible Church—had started running an antiabortion ad on TV that showed a black man hanging from a tree, Indians on a reservation, and Jewish Holocaust victims, the idea being that a woman deciding to have an abortion was the moral equivalent of racist murderers, those who massacred Indians, and Nazi genocidal psychopaths. The pastor of the church shrugged off criticism of the ad and told a newspaper reporter he planned to run it indefinitely.

That ad was stuck in my head while I was preparing this *Roe* v. *Wade* speech. It gave such a vivid depiction of the mentality of these so-called religious people. I knew I was going to have to say something about it. That morning was clear and sunny and cold. Chester sat with me at my kitchen table and helped me while I was writing. Then he and Oliver drove me to the Capitol. The right-to-lifers were going to be demonstrating and carrying on, and Oliver was concerned about my safety. He didn't want me parking and having to walk a long way. This way I could get out in front of the rotunda, and one of them could go in with me while the other parked the car.

"Look who's fighting the prochoice movement," I told the crowd after I got unlimbered a little. "A celibate, male-dominated church." I didn't actually mean the extremist fundamentalists were celibate; I wanted to get the Catholic hierarchy in there too. "We are talking about abortions," I said. "For hundreds of years black people had their freedom aborted, and the church said nothing! The way of life of Native Americans was aborted, and the church was silent! A whole race of people was eradicated in the Holocaust, and the church was silent!" It was an exaggeration, maybe, but not by much.

"These people should get over their love affair with the fetus. They all want to love little babies as long as they're in someone else's uterus. But they do not support welfare. They do not support Medicaid; they do not support good schools. They do not support the things that support children. They just want to take care of the fetus until it's born. And when it's born, they're ready to drop it and move on to getting somebody else born. That's a love affair. You can go and take it and drop it when you get finished with it. You don't have to worry about it. But with children, you've got to take care of them forever. With children it's not an affair; it's a marriage."

I was letting it all out. All my anger at the falseness and hypocrisy and the sitting in God's judgment seat. Which wasn't just words but meant thousands and thousands of girls every year in Arkansas consigned to being slaves for life in the kingdom of need, girls whose faces I saw with my own eyes every time I visited one of our clinics. Girls who lived in conditions I knew by heart, but these people didn't care to see. "These people," I told them, "are non-Christians with a slave driver mentality."

———

Tom Butler wasn't there for any of those *Roe* v. *Wade* speeches. But if he had been, those were times he would have been sweating bullets. The people on the extreme right had all their hackles up even before the first time I spoke at the rotunda. Afterward they were in a furious rage, which came out in every outlet they had, including the budget hearings that were going on. Pregnancy, according to some of the fundamentalists, was God's punishment for fornication. From that it followed that contraceptives were anti-God. School-based health services meant sex clinics and abortion mills. According to them, my arguments about how the clinics would provide children with badly needed health care were lies. We were using those arguments as a pretense so we could go in and perform abortions. Sex education meant teaching five-year-olds to have sex, just as years later in Washington I was accused of wanting to teach children how to masturbate. Of course only somebody that's really sick in the head could even think such things, and I'm not sure how many actually believed them. But those were the kinds of ideas that were flying around over what we were proposing. I never minded fighting about these things, but the atmosphere of hysteria and craziness about sex was enough to make your head spin. On occasion I'd catch myself daydreaming about the beautiful sanity of my old life in science.

I wasn't at all the hearings, only the ones where Tom thought it was important. One reason was that I had become a lightning rod. Too often the fight was not really about the issues but about me. All the antiabortion groups were testifying: the Right to Life, Arkansas Family Council, FLAG (Family, Life, America, God), and others. Sometimes we knew we had the votes and it was already taken care of, so it was best just to let them say what they had to say without getting involved. Other times it was a brawl, on occasion with one or another of the national leaders of these groups, who had been invited in to testify as a guest of the local chapter.

Sometimes that worked out well for us. Someone would be going on about sex clinics and abortions, and I'd say, "That's not what school-based clinics are about. They're about providing primary preventive health care in school where the children are—physical evaluations and dental care and counseling. We want to see the problems early so we can catch them early, treat them early, and take care of them and not let children suffer for years until it gets to be a chronic disease. Most of these children don't have a family doctor and never have any real health care."

And they'd say, "That's not what they're about."

And Knox Nelson would say, "Well, ma'am, Dr. Elders said that these were about health and keeping children healthy and doing physicals. Now what's wrong with that?"

"But that's not what they do. That's only a disguise they're using."

"Oh, what you're saying is Dr. Elders is lying? You don't live here. You don't know anything about this state. And you are going to tell us what Dr. Elders is going to do in a clinic that you don't know anything about?"

I remember one time Nelson got so mad at one right-to-life

leader that he slammed the table and said, "Ma'am, I told you I didn't want all of that stuff you're talking about. I asked you a specific question, and if you can't address that, then just shut it off."

But it didn't always work out in our favor either. Many of the legislators represented rural communities where there was a lot of fundamentalist feeling and not much knowledge of the real issues. So this was not by any stretch a one-way fight. We did get through the budget and health committee, but emotions were so high that the full legislature was still debating it the night of the deadline to close down the session.

Only about 30 percent of the health department budget actually came from state funds; the rest was from the federal government and private sources. But in Arkansas the legislature has to approve spending, even if it isn't from state money. Our total budget was for two hundred million dollars, of which we wanted authority to spend a million for school clinics, two thousand dollars of which was going to go for condoms. But that one-million-dollar authority and especially those two thousand dollars were threatening to drive the legislature and all the rest of us, including the governor, straight to distraction.

The problem was that on appropriation bills you need a 75 percent majority, which we had in the Senate, but it was close in the House, where twenty-five or twenty-six conservatives were holding up our entire budget in order to prevent approval of school-based clinics and condom distribution. By the time the last hours of the session started looming, the two houses had spent over two hundred thousand dollars' worth of their time fighting over two thousand dollars of condom money.

Tom Butler, Nancy Kirsch, and I were trying to shepherd things along from the governor's office in the Capitol, along with George Harper, the health department's general counsel. Governor Clinton was there too, and some of his staff, and messages were flying back and forth between the two houses and between us and the legislators, trying to find some compromise that we could live with and enough conservative representatives could vote for. Competing proposals were bouncing around like Ping-Pong balls.

At some point in the night Tom Butler said he thought I should go home and relax. Since he was the political expert, I did what he told me and drove home and got into bed. But I didn't relax. The phone kept ringing with different legislators calling me, especially our supporters in the Senate, like Nick Wilson and Jay Bradford, who wanted to hang tough and not give an inch to the House conservatives. It was getting late, and the senators were feeling their oats. They just knew the opposition was about to give it up, and I shouldn't agree to a thing they wanted.

I knew it was a mistake to come home, that we'd just end up getting our wires crossed. I knew it even before I picked up the phone and it was the governor, stomping mad. "Joycelyn! I was going to leave town this evening, and now I'm standing here fighting about your damned health bill! And we told you we were telling Bradford and them to vote for the bill modified like we said. And I told you I would take care of it. And then you went and told him somethin' else! And here I am suffering for your bill, and just what do you mean doin' that and I'm findin' it out from our people on the floor!" I mean, he was screaming. Just out of control.

I wasn't even quite sure what the mix-up was, so I called Tom and said, "Don't send me any more messages. I'm coming back." But by the time I got down there they had voted out the bill. When the media saw me coming, they crowded around and wanted to know if I would go on TV together with a right-to-life person, for the late news.

Then Tom pushed through and said, "It's all over. I think we got it. They said we can't use any state money, but we can have the clinics, and we can buy the condoms."

I said, "Tom, we've got two hundred million dollars, and the condoms cost two thousand. If we can't find two thousand dollars to buy condoms, we're going to need some new accountants."

Chapter 18

The Job's Available

❦

Bill Clinton got sputtering mad sometimes, but it was always a passing storm. Except one time when we didn't speak for three months over some funding the administration raised for education, none of which got allocated to our early-childhood programs though I lobbied Clinton's staff hard for it. Afterward I told him, "I just can't believe you are putting all that money into education and none of it where you can make the most difference." I was angry. Then he got angry that I hadn't gone to him personally about it and said some things he probably regretted, the result of which was that we weren't on speaking terms until months later, when Chester saw him someplace and said, "When are you and my sister going to get together and stop feuding?"

After that Clinton told me, "Anytime you have something you need to tell me, you find me. Okay? My people are instructed to get me. The state police, everybody. So if you need me, you just make sure you get me." I think he felt bad about what had happened. It was an important error.

That was our one episode of real anger in the six years I worked for Clinton in Arkansas. We weren't beer-drinking friends, but I was at the mansion now and then on business. He'd ask me to stop by before work or on my way home, and if there was breakfast or dinner, occasionally I stayed. Something would be going on, and he'd say, "We should talk. Why don't you come over and have coffee and doughnuts before I take Chelsea to school?" So it was pretty casual. But not the kind of casual where you just stop by and come in the back door.

Hillary traveled a lot, and on three or four occasions when I was there, Chelsea would be the hostess and serve cookies. This was starting when she was just a little thing, probably no more than five or six years old. Clinton was very involved with her life. Until he left Arkansas, he carried Chelsea to school and picked her up every day personally. He didn't just send a car; he went himself. I noticed that however busy he might be, he'd always feel he had to stop to help her do her homework.

Before the 1988 primaries Clinton asked if I thought he should run for President. I told him I didn't think so. I thought that it was a little late and that Bush was too strong anyway. I'm sure he was asking everyone in sight. I certainly wasn't someone whose advice he regularly sought on subjects other than health policy. But I do know that most people expected him to make that run, and it came as a big surprise when he said he wasn't going to. From what I could see, the decision had a lot to do with Chelsea. He thought she was too young and it was just not the right time for him to be away from her as much as he'd have to be.

So he didn't run, but of course he did give the famous nominating speech at the convention. I was in Washington, D.C., for a meeting of the FDA commission, at the Rockville Marriott, and I told all my friends, "You go home now. You are going to hear the most wonderful speech ever. You go home and you just listen to *my* governor." I really put on a brag show. I was very proud of Clinton. I had heard him speak a hundred times, and he was almost always superb. In Arkansas he probably never prepared a speech. He just got up and talked; he was a great extemporaneous speaker. I knew he had been working hard on the nominating speech; he had been talking about it a lot. So it figured to be showstopper.

Jesse Jackson went first and gave a gorgeous speech on the

great American quilt. Jesse was in his glory that night; it may have been the most moving piece of oratory he ever gave. But the whole time I was listening to him I was thinking, What a great preliminary. I couldn't wait to hear how Clinton was going to follow it.

But once Clinton did start speaking, he didn't stop. I was so embarrassed. I remembered he had said that Dukakis had gone over his speech and told him it was fine and that he should leave everything in. But thinking about it, Dukakis was probably too worried about his own speech to be much of a judge, especially since he himself wasn't a great speaker. He tended to be boring and go on, which is what Bill Clinton did that night. He's probably still kicking himself about it.

But that was one of the few political missteps I saw Clinton make. I was working closely with him on health issues, and he was good; he knew how to push those budgets. He didn't usually get up on the barricades himself. He didn't have to; I was doing enough talking for both of us. But he knew everything that was going on. We'd send the different elements over for his approval, and I'd brief him about the most significant programs. Then his people would go pat every back that wanted patting and twist every arm that required twisting.

I think that as health director maybe I surprised Bill Clinton some at first. He may not have expected me to focus my attention exactly the way I did, and he probably didn't anticipate the language I used. Then again, he could never have guessed how personal my involvement in this job was going to be. But whether he was surprised or not, I don't believe there was ever any real difference between us in our assessment of Arkansas's health needs.

Clinton quickly grasped the scope of the teenage pregnancy problem and its role in the cycle of poverty and despair. He knew Arkansas from top to bottom, and he understood the need to deliver health services to children. He didn't have to be told twice what the obstacles were either. He gave me completely free rein to go after these and other problems. As I soon learned, that was fundamentally different from the caution with which almost all governors handled their health departments. Teenage out-of-wedlock pregnancy was not an Arkansas phenomenon. Nor were AIDS and other STDs. But sexual issues made volatile politics, and in 1987 there weren't many governors willing to run that gauntlet.

Bill Clinton knew what he was doing. Some people said that he protected me because I staked out positions he couldn't and I took the heat for them. That may have been true to some extent; it wasn't something we ever talked about. But whether that was part of his concept of my role didn't concern me one way or the other. I knew what my priorities were, and I was ready to go after them regardless.

Clinton's hands-off approach ended up having broader consequences than either of us ever thought about. My fight with the antichoice, antieducation, anticondom fundamentalists was hot enough to begin attracting national attention. A local journalist named Steve Barnes wrote a piece about me that came out in *The New York Times.* Then *60 Minutes* and *MacNeil/Lehrer* decided I was controversial enough to do a story on. One result was that some additional interest got stirred up over school-based clinics and teenage pregnancy. The other was that every time I turned around somebody, especially other state health directors, was calling me about coming to speak.

Probably what spurred this attention more than the TV shows was when I was invited to speak at the annual convention of the American Public Health Association in New York. There were thirteen thousand people at that convention, including all the state health directors and the rest of the who's who in the national public health community. The meeting was held in the giant New York Hilton Grand Ballroom, and I was a panelist at one of many simultaneous groups that were going on. I was speaking about the effects of poverty on health, and I remember thinking in the middle of it that this was not the most inspiring performance I had ever given. But for some reason, either because they had seen me on television, or maybe I was just louder and more colorful than the other speakers who were on then, people started leaving the other groups and coming over to ours.

Once that started, the curiosity factor kicked in, and I found myself addressing a huge crowd instead of the hundred or so who had come to hear the panel on poverty. It was after this that I started being in real demand.

———

Meanwhile the Arkansas legislature had authorized ten school-based clinics, though it gave us only partial funding for them. Tom was working on the financial problem, figuring how we could cut back here and there and get along without something or put something else on hold till next session. I will never forget him coming into my office one day like a kid who just got the cookie jar opened saying, "Dr. Elders? We got the money." To this day I don't know where he got it all from, and I wasn't asking any questions either.

A little earlier we had put together a series of television spots on teenage pregnancy meant to heighten awareness of the problem. Channel 4, the local NBC affiliate, lumped all its public service announcement time for the year together so we could run advertisements aimed at teens, parents, and the business community. We put on panel discussions with doctors: four thirty-minute segments and then a series of one-minute, thirty-second, and fifteen-second spots that played throughout the day, strategically placed.

Now that we had the money, the next thing was to make sure we perked up some interest from the educators. We saw to it that all the districts in the state knew we were going to fund clinics fully for the first ten schools that applied. They wouldn't cost the schools that got them a cent. Our application criteria were based on need, but the first ten schools that applied and qualified would get the clinics.

The first step in the application process was for schools to get approval from their local boards. Then they had to guarantee space and meet a few other minimal provisions. Other than that, they were free to decide for themselves what services they wanted in their clinic. Of course I was hoping they would ask for family planning, including condom distribution. I was targeting our poorest districts, and we announced that preference would be given to schools with the highest teenage pregnancy rates.

Later some U.S. senators and right-wing spokespeople were going around claiming that school-based clinics were another awful example of the government forcing its secular, humanistic mores on people. The truth, which they all knew, was that the clinics were controlled locally from day one. Anything the local school committees wanted to exclude they could. Also, we set it up so a special board would help oversee each clinic. Our recommendation was that this board would include two people from the school, two local ministers, two people from the Arkansas judicial department, two parents, and two students. Plus, in any school that opted to include family planning services, only students who had consent forms signed by their parents were allowed to use them. If there was ever a more striking model of a government program under local control, I am not aware of it.

While the application process was going on, we actually had one school-based clinic up and running already, in Lakeview, a little town in the heart of the delta, Louise Dennis's territory. The high school there had approached us some time before through Joyce Gibson, one of Louise's career health care workers. This Lakeview school was 90-plus percent poor black, and three quarters of the senior girls either were pregnant or already had babies. "What can you do to help us here?" the principal asked Joyce. "We'll do whatever we have to; we'll even do condoms."

When we followed up, we found that the principal, the superintendent, and the board were serious about turning their situation around. We applied for a grant from Maternal Child Health in Washington and got funding for a pilot clinic. The federal money let us set Lakeview up as a more intensive program than we were going to be able to afford ourselves. The school provided two very nice rooms right next to the principal's office, and we had a full-time nurse practitioner and nurse's aide who did examinations and counseling and classroom teaching. A social worker was there several times a week, as were a nutritionist and a doctor. We did smoking and alcohol and drug counseling. Our dentist came in once a month to examine students, then went back to do repairs or make referrals. Besides him, the local dentists in nearby Helena set aside times when they would see kids on a pro bono basis, unless they had Medicaid, in which case we did the paper work for them. We also provided transportation, not just for the dentists but for other health services.

In the first screening, we found that 125 of the kids had significant dental problems. The medical screenings were even more sobering. We found hypertension and heart murmurs and a variety of other conditions. Maybe the worst part was the world of sexual abuse we uncovered and the widespread feeling among these young people that life was not worth living, which was connected directly with alcohol and drug use and early sexual activity. That led to our putting a psychological social worker in the school. We did home visits and worked with families and coordinated what we were doing with the department of human services. We engaged these problems with all the resources that grant gave us.

The first year our clinic was up and running the pregnancy rate at Lakeview High School went to zero, which was where it stayed for four years. After that we had to back off because the noise over family planning and distributing condoms got so loud. Needless to say, the rate immediately started up again.

Lakeview worked beautifully. The school was behind it, and the churches and community supported the programs. We tracked everything and learned which interventions worked well and which didn't and why. We couldn't have asked for a better pilot.

Lakeview was like a smaller Marianna, the town whose public health clinic was in the old jailhouse with the hanging room. Marianna was a place I really wanted to go; it met all the criteria. The pregnancy rate was high; the poverty rate was high; medical services were scant. It needed a clinic as badly as anyone in the state. I was familiar with the school to a certain extent. Oliver used to go down and play them every Christmas, and I sometimes went with him. Also, the new superintendent there was a woman I knew, and she convinced me the school really wanted to do this.

So I started doing the groundwork. The Deltas invited me down, and I gave a talk in one of the bigger black churches. I met with the Kiwanis and the Chamber of Commerce and spoke to the students and faculty at the high school. I probably made four or five visits to Marianna, which was what I had begun to do wherever we were looking to set up a clinic. The school board was going to make the decision, so the community had to be well informed and its questions had to be answered. I thought everything in Marianna was about ready to go.

But when I arrived for the open meeting where the school board was going to vote, I knew I was in trouble the moment I walked in the door. The big room was packed with people, just wall to wall, and maybe 90 percent of them were white—this in a city where 99 percent of the public high school students were black. Like many places in Arkansas, after the Supreme Court had outlawed school segregation, Marianna's white community had set up private all-white schools and left the public schools to the black community. But the school board was still mostly white, and the political and business establishments and landowners were almost all white. These people and their supporters were the ones packed in wall to wall, along with a scattering of handpicked blacks. I didn't know they were handpicked at first, but I understood the instant they opened their mouths to speak.

That happened directly after I gave my presentation. The first black woman got up and told me, "I don't know what you're down here talking about. God don't want us not to have children. That's why when these older folks don't want to have children, God puts the babies in the children." That was how it started. "My daughter's never going to take birth control pills because babies are like the trees in the forest. God wants them there." The level of discussion rarely climbed higher than that. Sex education and birth control and abortion were one and the same. One led to the next, and they all were an abomination. I recognized early on that a lot of the folks there were from FLAG. The ignorance was enough to make you cry tears. "We know what we want for our town, and you're just trying to prevent black people from growing their race." That was from another black woman. Let me tell you, they made sure that they had their right set of people there.

It could have been that in 1988 Marianna's history still bore too heavily on the town. In the sixties Marianna had been the site of one of Lyndon Johnson's big War on Poverty programs. A cooperative health clinic had been set up and had become the center of all sorts of services: not just health care, but food stamps, and voter registration, and legal aid—the whole ball of wax, all of it helped along by a big group of Vista volunteers. I knew something about that. I had been there too on a couple of occasions, sent down by the medical school to work in the clinic.

When that War on Poverty program got under way, the town of Marianna went into a kind of political culture spasm. Nothing much had changed there since post-Reconstruction times, and now this health center and so on was beginning to educate people and make them aware of their situation. It just enraged the power structure of the day. They thought these outsiders were "exciting our niggers," as the newspaper very picturesquely put it. They were getting them worked up. There was racial tension and unrest. Blacks boycotted stores, and Joan Baez came down to sing protest songs. I don't think it's a time Marianna looks back on with much pride.

I don't recall exactly how that period ended, but while it lasted, it wasn't pretty. And the whole thing more or less had started with the health center. All that had happened more than twenty years back. But listening to the anger and fear at that school board hearing made me think that those emotions hadn't run their course even yet. The motion to have a school-based clinic was voted down, of course. By a big margin.

By contrast, one of the places that voted yes for a clinic was Lincoln, a town of fifteen hundred or so in northwest Arkansas near the Oklahoma border. That area is almost 100 percent white and as conservative as anywhere in the state. So it surprised some people that the townspeople were so anxious to have a clinic there, though not me. I had visited that area when I did my tour of health department clinics the previous November, and I knew what conditions many of the people up there were living in. Lincoln High School, it turned out, had thirteen girls in the senior class, and many of them either were or had been pregnant.

———

Oliver's mother, Leona, was a dynamo. She was one of those schoolteachers who were so intent on doing the best for their students that they kept up on and tried out every promising development that came along. Even then she had tons more energy than just teaching first and second grade could absorb. She set up and ran a Head Start program in De Witt, established another program to feed children living in poverty, and made the local shoe factory give her shoes for those who needed them. There was an old school for black children down there that had been closed for years, and Leona and Prof, Oliver's dad, had got the town to give it to them. They fixed up the gym and put in a program of activities. They opened a day-care center and a center to distribute goods to poor people. Leona was a force of nature with a heart you couldn't measure.

After we had Eric and Kevin, I told her, "You know, these are your grandchildren, and I expect you to keep them at least a month every summer."

Leona's answer to that was: "Well, all right!" And every summer she'd start planning what to do. She took them to Disney World and Six Flags and anywhere else she thought they might enjoy going.

I'd tell her, "Really, Leona, you don't need to—" and she'd say, "No, this is my month, and I want them."

In 1988 Leona was eighty-seven, and Prof was ninety-one. For the previous year or so Leona had been failing. Prof tried to keep it a secret, but Oliver and I knew what was happening. Leona had come up to Little Rock for knee surgery and had stayed with us for several months while she was convalescing.

It was obvious then that she was in the first stages of Alzheimer's. She mainly sat on the porch and looked out over the lake.

Once she went back to De Witt, she started deteriorating quickly, and at the same time Oliver's dad was getting sick and wasn't able to take care of her. We did everything we could to help from a distance, but finally in September we decided to bring them up to our house. We hired a woman to help out during the day, which was fine, but by then Leona had given up sleeping at night. In her agitation she'd go from room to room, turning on lights and anything else that could be turned on. After one close call with the kitchen stove, we took all the knobs off that and did whatever else we could to make the house safe.

One night I heard noises, and when I got up to check things out, I found Oliver's dad trying to get Leona back to bed. He had not been feeling well; in the past week Oliver had taken him to the doctor two or three times. I said, "Prof, what are you doing up?"

"I'm trying to get her back," he said, "so she won't bother anybody."

"Well," I said, "there's nobody in this house for her to bother except me and her son and her grandson. All you're going to do is get yourself sick. You get up from there right now, and you get in that bed and go to sleep. I mean it."

The next morning our home care person came in, and Oliver and I left for work. She fixed breakfast for Oliver's dad, then went back to the bedroom to take care of Leona. After she had bathed and dressed her, she brought Leona into the kitchen and found Oliver's dad slumped down over the table, dead of a heart attack.

Of course Oliver and I had talked about this kind of possibility, not just for Prof and Leona, but for my parents too. Basically we had concluded that when the time came, he would decide what should be done in regard to his parents, I would decide about mine, and whatever one of us decided the other would support. As long as Oliver's dad was able to be a companion to Leona, we didn't have any real question about what to do. But when Prof died, it came to a head. Oliver may have considered a nursing home arrangement briefly, but when it came down to it, he wasn't anywhere near able to bring himself to send her off somewhere.

With Leona we saw the full gamut of Alzheimer's, from slight disorientation to hyperactivity to something near vegetativeness. At first our helper was coming in for six or seven hours a day, but as Leona became more disabled, we had to change things around. Before long I developed a routine that I could get done in thirty minutes before I had to leave for work. I'd strip the bed, give her a bath, then have her coffee ready and put her on the commode. While she was there, I'd get her orange juice and fix her oatmeal and Ensure, a balanced nutrition product. By the time I had Leona in a chair eating, our helper was coming in the door and I was on my way out.

While Leona was able to help some, I could take care of her by myself. But when it got to the point where she couldn't, Oliver was always there to give me a hand with her. If somebody had told me a few months earlier that I'd have to make extra time in my schedule to take care of a sick person, I'd have laughed out loud. But necessity has a way of teaching you to accommodate.

Starting back when I was a resident, I had worked a day a week as the medical superviser in a nursing home, which at that point meant for twenty-six or twenty-seven years. Usually I was at the home on a Saturday or Sunday to review the records, take care of anyone who was sick, sign orders, and discuss cases with the full-time nurse practitioners. Over the years I had acquired a lot of experience with elderly patients. I was used to taking care of them. But even with that, it was hard dealing with this woman who had been such a powerful figure with so loving a nature, whose beautiful personality now was fading away along with her physical and mental abilities.

As she drifted farther off, I think I came to see Leona less as the mother-in-law who had done so many wonderful things for my family and others and more as a patient. But that's never completely possible. Up to the end—Leona lived until 1993—

even when everything else was gone, she remembered me and always wanted "Joyce" for whatever might have flashed momentarily across her mind. I know how extremely hard those years were for Oliver and me, despite my lifetime experience of caring for patients. It gave me a feeling for the heroic effort made by families that don't have that kind of background to draw on and don't have the financial resources that helped us to cope. When I started the fight to expand Arkansas's in-home health care services, I had a pretty good feel for what was needed, and why.

I fought that particular fight right up till I left for Washington, six years later. By then we were providing in-home care in all but a few counties, primarily to our frail and elderly, though also for children and AIDS patients. We had expanded from a half-million-dollar-a-year in-home operation to a twenty-eight-million-dollar-a-year service, the money coming from Medicare, Medicaid, and insurers. It was a win/win situation: our costs of three or four thousand dollars per patient per year compared with twelve to eighteen thousand for putting them in a nursing home. The patients liked it better; their families liked it better. The legislature was sold on the savings and on the improvement in life for their constituents.

The only folks who didn't like it were the home health businesses. They wanted to skim off the cream and take care of the easy ones, leaving us the ones in rural areas who were poor, had no insurance, and were difficult to pay for. They didn't feel that they should have to compete with the state in providing home health, that we should send them all the paying ones and we could take care of the nonpaying ones. I just told them they were as crazy as worms. In the end they were strong enough only in six counties to keep us out. I think that if the health department had done nothing else while I was director, our in-home program would have made those years worthwhile.

As the toll from AIDS grew, we also set up in-home hospice care. We were putting tremendous effort into AIDS education, though that was an endless struggle because of these people who knew it was immoral to talk about sex in schools but never could explain how we might educate about AIDS prevention without referring to it. So we were working hard to get AIDS education into schools and to persuade the churches to start up their own education programs. That was on the prevention side. At the same time we were working with the churches to help provide home care for AIDS patients who were terminally ill.

One event that helped galvanize the mainstream religious community was when the minister of one of the largest churches in Little Rock contracted HIV through a blood transfusion. His talk about that to his congregation moved many people and spurred a lot of newspaper and radio coverage. After that a significant group of churches got involved in AIDS work.

What the churches did mainly was provide volunteers. Our public health nurses went in to administer IV fluids and do pain management while church members went to sit and read and talk or maybe provide meals or transportation to family members if they needed it or go shopping for them. We urged the churches to adopt people they knew with terminal AIDS and help us help them spend their last weeks or days in as much comfort and dignity as possible. I hired a full-time person to serve as liaison with the churches. We worked hard to mobilize them to be our partner in this.

We had some real successes with the churches, but the one minister who absolutely exemplified service to the community was Reverend Bill Robinson of Hoover United Methodist. He was and still is the best grass-roots organizer I know. Hoover Methodist runs a huge day-care center, a model AIDS program, a drug addiction center that sees a hundred people a day, a shelter for battered and homeless women, and a bunch of other things. William Robinson is far from being the kind of polished, smooth religious person you often see on the TV. Instead he lives the Gospel. His church does what all churches should be about. He goes down into the trenches every day, doing what he can to alleviate suffering. He preaches the sermon of hope. I used to go down to Hoover and listen to him sometimes. "You are important," he tells his congregation. "God has not forgotten you. God will never forget you."

I put Reverend Robinson on one of the health department boards and used him in every forum I possibly could. We ended up sending him to speak on AIDS all over the country. His AIDS program became a national model, and then the person who was over my organization, Sonya Hunt, was hired by the Centers for Disease Control to coordinate its AIDS prevention effort with church-sponsored programs.

I might have been concentrating on teenage pregnancy, but I took Lisbeth Schorr's lesson on multiple strategies to heart. Over the next five years I expanded our children's health screening services, improved our early-childhood immunizations from 30 to 64 percent, and put in place the kind of tracking system you need if you want to get the immunization rate up permanently. I was out fighting for early-childhood enrichment programs, the ones I had the set-to with Governor Clinton about. I supported the drug education that was being sponsored by Robert Wood Johnson, even though its focus was on treatment and I wanted the resources used for education and prevention. Interestingly there was no trouble getting the drug education program into schools. I didn't hear any of the conservatives shouting that drug education would lead to increased drug use, even though every time you cared to listen somebody or other was going off on how sex education was certain to open the floodgates of youthful immorality.

One program we got money for that didn't work out the way I wanted was college scholarships. I fought hard to get college education money for kids living in poverty. Some people might have thought that was a stretch for the health department, but in my mind there was plenty of justification. It wasn't just that you couldn't keep ignorant people healthy; it was that so many of our children were members of what in my speeches I was calling the 5H Club: hungry, helpless, homeless, hugless, hopeless. Those high schoolers in Lakeview who didn't know if life was worth living weren't an anomaly. They saw no hope of ever getting out of the conditions they were born into. I knew all I needed to know about that, and I thought that it wouldn't cost us much to inject some hope into these hopeless lives by telling good students they would be able to go to college.

My proposal was that Arkansas students who had a B average, showed good citizenship, had their principals' recommendations, and couldn't afford college should have their tuition paid at a state institution. I wanted something that would help give poor kids who were striving to do well some optimism about the future. In the end the legislature passed a bill along those lines, except it added more academic criteria and made the stipends independent of need. So in effect it did nothing except just get the rich richer and the poor poorer.

So I lost that one, but there were other areas where we succeeded. We established a women's health agenda with programs to alleviate violence against women and child abuse; we set up a rape crisis center, women's shelters, a drug rehabilitation program for women. We improved our family planning counseling and provided Norplant contraceptive implants for poor women who wanted it. We brought up our prenatal-care levels, improved the WIC program of food supplements to needy mothers with children, and increased our mammogram screenings. At the same time we computerized the health system and made a great effort to attract doctors to rural areas that didn't have any, getting seventeen of them. All that happened in a period of three legislative sessions, six years. We were busy, Tom and I and everyone else. The health department grew from fifteen hundred to twenty-six hundred employees and seemed like it was bursting with energy. Whatever lightning we might have been striking, those health workers were the thunder behind it.

Most of our accomplishments came from hard work behind the scenes and building bridges with the legislators. But my last fight in the Capitol, just before I left for Washington, didn't go well at all. In a way you might say it was good preparation for what was to come.

In 1993 I was looking for a way to set up a children's trust fund that would provide ongoing support for health education, early-childhood education, health coverage for below-poverty-line children, and other screening and treatment services. After looking at a number of possible money sources, I decided the best way to fund this trust would be by increasing the tax on cigarettes. That made sense because the cigarette tax was the lowest it had been in over thirty-five years. In 1955 the tax had been 23 percent of the package price. Now it was under 20 percent. But there were two problems with that. One was that each year the tobacco lobby gave a load of money to Arkansas politicians, and the second was that Governor Jim Guy Tucker, Bill Clinton's successor, had persuaded the legislature to pass a small tax increase on cigarettes not very long before.

That was to shore up Arkansas's Medicaid program, which had gone bankrupt. The state funded only 25 percent of Medicaid; the rest was federal. But the state fund had run out of money. To bail it out, Governor Tucker had called a special session and gotten it to pass a tax on soda pop and cigarettes, which did the job, even though the cigarette tax was only nine cents a pack. But Tucker had had to fight his head off even for that, and the general impression was that in the end the tobacco industry gave it to him as a kind of sop.

I felt that nine cents was meaningless. I needed thirty-two cents on top of that, which was what my proposal was for. Tom tried to dissuade me from making this fight. He believed it didn't have a snowball's chance and we'd just be killed. But I knew I could present an overwhelmingly strong case, and I also thought that shame would be my ally. Smoking cost a fortune in health expenses, and smoking-related diseases were the state's second leading cause of death. Taking some tobacco money to support children's health had a lot of merit to it. I thought that making a moral issue of that might do us a world of good in the committee. I was calling the trust fund Children First.

I prepared thoroughly for that hearing. I lined up witnesses from the American Heart Association, the Cancer Society, the American Lung Association, and an array of other medical experts, maybe ten or twelve of them altogether. I also had cancer patient witnesses, a couple of whom had had laryngectomies from smoking-induced throat cancer and spoke through boxes, which had a persuasive effect. I don't think in my entire public health career I had ever made a more powerful presentation.

I should have been warned, though, when I saw that the other side didn't present a single witness. That's how sure of themselves they were. As far as they were concerned, they had passed this little piecemeal tax before, which was all they needed to soothe their consciences about doing what the lobbyists told them. I must say that Tom had tried to prepare me for what was going to happen. He said he didn't expect us to get more than four or five votes. I don't know if he believed that or if he was trying to put a kind face on his realism. When the vote was called, after no real debate to speak of, we got two votes. That's my memory of it. Tom says it was one.

When I left that committee room after the vote, I was fit to be tied. Then right outside in the corridor I was corralled by a bunch of media people sticking microphones and cameras at me. Someone asked what my reaction was and what kind of message I thought the vote sent. Now just a short time before this the legislature had granted some special tax favors to the racetrack at Hot Springs. It had also given relief to the alcohol industry. "Your legislators," I started saying, "your legislators just sold your children out to the gamblers, to the tobacco industry, and to the whiskey dealers." Right then two of the committee members walked by not a yard from where we were standing. "And there they are." I pointed and waggled my finger at them. "There go two of them now!" The cameras swung around, which startled them a little. I think Tom was trying to get me away from there; he tried to keep me out of these frays if he could. He was saying it was all right; I'd live to fight another day. I told him he could bet money I would.

———

That was in March, at the very end of the 1993 session. Actually we had already done pretty well with getting our budget through the legislature. I didn't mind making people mad, which I knew this cigarette tax proposal was going to do, but I figured there was no point in upsetting them before they had voted out the rest of what we wanted. I also knew that I might as well go out swinging for something that was really important. Bill Clinton was now President, and several months earlier he had nominated me for surgeon general. My confirmation hearings were coming up soon, and this was pretty much the last thing I was going to be doing as director of health in Arkansas.

Actually, for some time now I had been paying almost as much attention to national health policy as I was to state problems. The Bush administration had invited me to serve on its committee that was developing health reform legislation, which I had been doing for almost two years. I had also been elected president of ASTHO, the Association of State and Territorial Health Officials, and was in constant touch with other state health directors on what was going on around the country and on all the significant health legislation in the works. We had our own national office in Washington and were working on various major projects, like the big Healthy People 2000 initiative and revamping national health data management to make the data sets accessible and relevant to each state, so we wouldn't have two- and three-year lags in comparing statistics.

I had really started getting to know the state health directors in 1988 during our first teenage pregnancy debates. I had begun getting speaking invitations from them then, and over the years they had just snowballed. Sometimes I addressed their legislatures about bills, sometimes their health or education departments, sometimes public forums if there was a big health debate going on. By 1993 I could count the states I hadn't spoken in on one hand.

Typically the directors wanted me to talk about teenage pregnancy and school-based clinics, which I could do without the political constraints they or their governors might be under. I spoke in unlikely places, like Utah, where they didn't like to admit they had a teenage pregnancy problem, except that they did have one. And Alabama, where the governor wasn't supportive but his wife was, and maybe he was too underneath but he wanted to get himself reelected. I think they also knew that I wasn't going to be shy about zapping the Christian Coalition types, who were always picketing and making noise. It was a lot easier for someone like me to let them have it, then leave, than it was for the local health directors who were going to have to live there afterward. I say it was lots easier for me, mainly because I didn't have to worry about them in Arkansas, where Bill Clinton was my constituency of one for six years. But when I went to Washington, of course, I brought that history along with me.

—

During the 1992 presidential election I didn't work on Clinton's campaign. According to law, I couldn't unless I resigned first. But I was doing a lot of speaking around the country, as usual, and I did talk about the health improvements we had managed in Arkansas under his leadership. Clinton never spoke to me about the race, but he knew I was out there. He'd say, "Well, you're everywhere. Every time I go somewhere people are coming up and telling me that you were just there."

On election night I went to bed early, but I got up at about two or three o'clock and turned the television on. All the votes weren't in, but Clinton was ahead, and it looked good. The next day Little Rock was like New York on New Year's. It seemed like everyone in the state was walking around downtown, smiling and congratulating each other.

I was as happy as a clam myself, but going to Washington wasn't part of any plans I had. I was really enjoying being health director, and I had been elected president of the state health officers only a couple of months back. Clinton had never mentioned anything to me about the future, but Jim Guy Tucker, the lieutenant governor who was going to fill out his term, had already asked me to stay on. I was either going to do that or maybe go back to the university. I hadn't decided which.

The first inkling I had about something else didn't come from Clinton, it came from Louis Sullivan, George Bush's secretary of health and human services. I knew Louis well. He had been president of Morehouse College Medical School before his Cabinet appointment, and in past years he had tried hard to get me to take the pediatric chairmanship there. More recently we had worked together on President Bush's health reform legislation.

One day completely out of the blue Louis called and said, "Joycelyn, if anybody ever asks, this conversation never happened. I'll deny it if you say it did. But I've heard you might be appointed the next health and human services secretary. If you are appointed, I've got a lot of things that will be very helpful to you."

About a week later Clinton called me at work and asked if I could stop by the governor's mansion that evening on my way home. I said I would, but when I got there, the place was in a turmoil. People were just kind of rummaging around everywhere. I saw Mickey Kantor and Warren Christopher and a lot of those people coming in and out. So I just sat down and chatted with some of the help and a few of the campaign people who were floating around until finally Clinton came out and said could I come up into the library.

When we got up there by ourselves, we talked a little about the election; he was still glowing from it. Then he said, "Joycelyn, I'd like for you to be the surgeon general. Would you consider that?" I was a little taken aback. I didn't know that I even wanted to be secretary.

"Why in the world would I want to be the surgeon general?" I said. "I've got a better job than that already."

"Well," he said, "I just think you could do a lot for the country."

"Governor, I've got more influence now being president of the state and territorial health officers than I'd ever have as surgeon general. And I've got twenty-six hundred people here in Arkansas. Besides, the surgeon general's term isn't up. I can't be appointed. You already have a surgeon general."

"No," he said. "The job's available. I've been assured Novello's going to resign and I can make the appointment."

"I'm not sure I'm interested," I said. "I feel the real job is being secretary. As far as I know the surgeon general doesn't have any power, and I've already got all the prestige and influence I can use."

"Well, let me think about it," he said. "I'll call you tomorrow."

Chapter 19

Signing On

❧❦❧

When I came home that night and told Oliver, he said, "Well, Sug, is that what you want to do, go to Washington?"

"No," I told him, "I don't really think so. But what am I going to say to Clinton?"

"If you don't want to do it," Oliver said, "just tell him. But you know, if you do want to, I think we have to talk about what I'm going to do up there."

So we discussed that some because it was a problem. Each of us had been turning down offers for years because they didn't make sense for the other one, and Oliver wasn't any more ready to retire than I was.

Clinton called the next morning. He had been assured that Antonia Novello was going to resign, he said, so that wasn't a concern. "I'd really like you to take the job," he told me. "I think you're the perfect person for it. As far as the secretary goes, I'm going to ask someone else to take that." Then he said, "You know, I've been thinking about Oliver too. I'd like for him to be over the President's Commission on Physical Fitness and Sports. Why don't we set up a time for you to come over and talk again?"

I gave serious consideration to not accepting. Other than visibility, the job didn't have that much going for it. Becoming surgeon general would mean a huge disruption in our lives for something that just wasn't that attractive. On the other hand, the state health directors all were urging me to take it. They would have rather I'd been offered the secretary's job, as I would have myself, since that was where the policy making was. But as surgeon general I'd have the prominence to draw attention to the agendas we'd been working on together practically since I became director.

In that time I had built a lot of bonds not just with the directors but with practically all the other public health groups too. I had friendships and contacts all over the country, which gave me a ready-made grass-roots network. My whole time as health director I had been speaking out on issues other public health officials couldn't talk about because they didn't have the leverage. But if I went to Washington, I'd be able to bring them real leverage. The surgeon general might not have much else, but she does have the bully pulpit. I'd have visibility like I never had.

While that wasn't totally compelling, it had its attractions. The job for Oliver was also tempting. Clinton was offering him the executive directorship of the Council on Sports and Fitness, which was known for its celebrity chairpeople, like Arnold Schwarzenegger and Jackie Joyner-Kersee. That was an important position that Oliver thought he'd really be able to handle well. If he was going to give up coaching, this was something he wouldn't mind doing it for.

Chester put his two cents in too. When he thought I might be deciding against it, he suggested I look in the Book of Jonah. In his opinion, God was calling me to Washington the same way He called Jonah to Nineveh. Personally I wasn't so sure. If He was calling me, how come He was talking about it to Chester?

Even my mother had an opinion. She had had a soft spot in her heart for Clinton ever since he came to Bernard's funeral. "You need to go on up there and help him," she told me on the telephone. "I saw him on TV the other night, and he just looked pitiful."

In the end I made up my mind to do it. I liked Clinton a lot personally; besides, I felt a loyalty to him. If he was asking me to do this, it would have been real hard to turn him down. Plus, I knew he'd be moving in the right direction on health care, and of course a major health overhaul was going to be in the works, so there was a chance to be involved in that.

Then there were the health directors, from whom I was getting a real ground swell of encouragement along with suggestions about programs I ought to try to get put under my jurisdiction. Although the surgeon general is a four-year statutory appointment, the office is under the jurisdiction of the secretary of health and human services and has no policy- or grant-making powers. As surgeon general you are chief of the Commissioned Corps, a federal health corps of six thousand plus that serves as the nation's medical shock troops. Beyond that you have the honor of being called the nation's top doctor, and you have a ready-made platform to give speeches from. For historical reasons the surgeon general also gets to wear a three-star admiral's uniform. But that's it.

So I began negotiating to have some policy input, directly with Clinton, who at the same time was talking about it with Donna Shalala, his nominee for HHS secretary. I didn't know Shalala at all, other than having heard that she was a friend of Hillary's. But it didn't seem as if she was putting up any unreasonable obstacles to what I was asking, which I took as a good sign for our future relationship.

During those discussions I was also on the phone a number of times with Everett Koop. Koop was friendly and helpful, telling me about the office and the problems he had had and what he thought I might do to build the job up to something more like what it had been before Richard Nixon had stripped a lot of its responsibilities. Clinton seemed to welcome the idea in principle, and before we were finished talking, he agreed also to appoint me deputy assistant secretary with responsibility for minority health, women's health, adolescent health, and family planning. That was announced along with my appointment as surgeon general on December 20.

When he and I finally sat down together in the mansion after everything had been settled, I said, "Governor, when you asked me to be your health director, you didn't know anything about me. But if you do this, you will know exactly what you are getting."

"Yeah," he said, "I know, Joycelyn. I think you'll be terrific. All I want is for you to do for the country what you've done for Arkansas."

"You know I tend to say what I think."

"I know that for sure," he said.

———

The day after the announcement I called Antonia Novello to talk with her about the job and to discuss how she wanted to handle the transition. To my considerable surprise she told me she didn't know anything about a transition. She didn't know she was being replaced, and she hadn't given any thought to resigning. As far as she was concerned, it was a four-year appointment, and she was still on the job.

Novello sounded embarrassed and a little angry. For myself, I was mortified. I told her I was sorry, I thought it all had been taken care of. I apologized, thinking, Let me just leave this alone.

It turned out later that Novello was starting to negotiate about her next appointment. Toni Novello was a professional Commissioned Corps officer who had been appointed surgeon general out of the ranks. Now that she had been the head of the Commissioned Corps, she wanted to take another position commensurate with her experience, instead of just going back to where she had been before, which of course she was right to want.

When we got friendly later on, I told her that was what I would have done too. "You just let me know what you want to do," I told her. "Tell me when you want to leave and when you think you've got everything lined up, so I can plan for my family."

"All right, Joycelyn," she said. "I think I'll have my assignment by the end of June, so I'll submit my resignation effective June thirtieth."

"That's wonderful," I said. "I'll tell the President we can go ahead on July first."

That was how come my confirmation didn't get to the Senate until July 1993, even though I was nominated along with the President's Cabinet in December after the election. But I didn't wait till July to start going to Washington. One of the first items on Clinton's agenda was health care reform, and shortly after the inauguration I found myself on one of the committees that were being set up. Before I began my commuting, though, a strange and terrible thing happened in Little Rock.

———

It was probably seven or eight years now that Nina, the girl I had been foster mother to, had moved out of the house. We were still in touch once in a while, although we didn't see each other too frequently anymore. I knew she had been living with a young man for quite a long time out in West Little Rock, the same one she had taken up with when she first moved out. He was from a pretty good family, but we heard that he had been in trouble with the law on occasion and that he had gotten her into trouble too. I knew their circumstances were pretty rugged. At some point Nina had told me they were planning to get married.

Sometime in late November Nina came by the house and stayed over for a couple of days. She and her young man had set a date for the wedding, she said, and she was looking to buy a wedding dress. She already had a really pretty one picked out, but she didn't have enough money for it. Did I have eight hundred dollars I could give her?

"No, I don't," I said. "If you need things, I don't mind helping you out. I don't mind giving you the money to buy a stove or a refrigerator, but I'm not going to spend any eight hundred dollars for a wedding dress, not especially when you've been with this man for eight years." I didn't know what she could have been thinking. She knew me well enough to know that the practical part of me was not about to invest in a wedding dress when she didn't have a refrigerator in her apartment.

Not too long after that I got a call from Nina at my office. Her voice was thin and choked. She sounded scared. She was calling from jail, she said. The police had picked her up on a drug charge and were holding her on ten thousand dollars' bail. Was there any way I might be able to put up the bond? As soon as I hung up, I called Oliver and told him what had happened. He went right over to the bank, then down to the jail to get her out.

Nina stayed with us for a day or so. Then her boyfriend came to pick her up. We knew they were going back to where they were living in West Little Rock. We had to know because of the bond. I was positive Nina wasn't planning to go running off anywhere.

A couple of weeks later Oliver and I were sitting at the table having coffee. He was reading the paper, and suddenly he blurted out, "Sug, look at this. Is this Nina?" The article was reporting a double homicide way out on Airport Road. Two people, a young man and a young woman, had been found shot to death in their car. The man was Nina's fiancé; the young woman was Nina. The police had no clues (nor did they ever find any).

The funeral was a few days later, down in Nina's hometown below Hot Springs. Oliver tried hard to convince me not to go, and when Chester came by, he added himself to that argument. They thought that Nina's mother and father would probably not have themselves under control. After their history with Nina they'd need to take their guilt out on somebody, and if I showed up there, I'd be the one they'd take it out on. I was so distraught, though, that I didn't care. I was going to go down there and be there and talk to them. Oliver was angry enough to spit. He thought I was really going to put myself in danger. So did Chester. That was a real backwoods all-white place, and emotions were bound to be high. "I know more about this kind of thing than you do," Chester was saying. "I've seen it! Don't you dare go down there!"

The way it ended up, Chester went with me. The paper said the funeral was going to be at ten, so I gave us some extra time since I had never been there and I knew her mother didn't live in town, but back in the country. I had her address. The father lived down there as well, and I know I had his address at one time too, but I couldn't seem to dig it up. Anyway, I figured we'd go to the church where it was supposed to be, and I'd see them there.

Well, when Chester and I got to the church, it turned out the funeral was set for one, not ten, like the paper said. So I made Chester drive over to the mother's house, which required a lot of driving around and looking. When we did finally get there, the people in the house saw us and came out before we had even gotten up to the door: the mother, an older woman who turned out to be the grandmother, and a bunch of others, all of them angry as hornets. The mother was bawling, "You should never have done that! This would have never happened if you hadn't gotten her out of jail! You killed her!"

And Chester was saying, "Joycelyn, let's go."

I was trying to explain, but all I could hear was "Why did you do it? Why did you get her out?"

And Chester was saying in my ear, "You don't talk rational sense to people who aren't rational. Now let's get out of here." So we left. I made Chester try to find the father's house, but we weren't able. We didn't stay for the funeral.

———

In February health reform got under way seriously, and I began flying up to Washington two days a week. I had been assigned to the committee on the underserved and poor, one of fifteen committees that were set up to develop plans on different elements of the health care problem. Each committee was supposed to work by itself. Ira Magaziner, a kind of business and social policy consultant, was appointed to coordinate and integrate everything, working mainly with Donna Shalala, now newly confirmed as HHS secretary, and Hillary Clinton.

Hillary had a lot of prominence, but it looked to me like everybody thought she was much more involved than she really was. She was doing a lot of work outside the task force, in terms of speeches and public relations and such, but she didn't seem to be spending any time around the committees. I don't think I ever saw her.

It might have gone better if she had been around more, at least as far as how things were organized. Other people might have had different impressions, but from the start mine was that the organization of the health reform task force was a sorry mess. I would fly up from Little Rock for committee meetings and find people milling around wondering where to go and what the agenda was. One Friday night I flew up for a special Saturday meeting that was supposed to be important, but when the time came, we didn't have a room to meet in. Some of us were sitting on the steps in the middle of the hall—this was in the Old Executive Office Building—and others were just roaming around. Nobody seemed to know where to go, what to do, or what it was about. A lot of those kinks eventually got worked out. But I was never impressed in my group that we were quite well enough organized to work methodically through the problems and develop a plan that was what it should have been.

What also surprised me were the people involved in the committees. Many of them seemed to be mid-level government bureaucrats. Others had worked on the campaign or were even doctors who knew something about one aspect of medicine or another. But there weren't a lot of people who were versed in health policy or experienced at getting things done in the health world. I couldn't imagine who might have come up with this mix or what they had in mind.

Mostly it just left me wondering, but sometimes it went far beyond that. At one point I was scheduled to give a breakfast talk on the reform program to a high-level group of health writers, editors, and power brokers, with a scattering of senators and representatives thrown in. My cospeaker was going to be Gail Wilensky, who had been in charge of the Bush administration's health reform efforts. I had been involved in those, so I knew Gail. She was a crackerjack, a highly accomplished person for whom I had tremendous respect.

Carol Rasco of the White House staff had me come into

Washington the night before so I could be thoroughly briefed; this was an event I had to be especially well prepared for. But when my briefers showed up, the main one turned out to be a medical student at Harvard and the other was a lobbyist of some sort. I couldn't believe my eyes. I'm sure the briefer was a bright young man, but he had all the depth of understanding on health care that you'd expect a student to have. In the end I thought, Well, I better talk on something I know about, so I focused my talk on the problems of adolescent health and the need to move from a sick care system to a preventive health care system.

That went just fine, for what it was. Gail Wilensky gave an insightful overview of the entire Bush health plan. I was just shocked that they would have sent a student to brief me about this. Thinking back on it, I still find it shocking. And it wasn't some isolated incident. The health care reform team was regularly sending out people who didn't know a thing about medicine to talk to major medical groups about health issues and reform policies.

Sometimes it seemed the decisions those in charge were making about people were nothing more than plain, willful stupidity. They seemed to be purposefully avoiding people who had a track record of making things happen in health. Instead they would invite a doctor someone happened to meet in South Carolina who happened to be friends with somebody else. They did not want to talk to the state health directors, which amazed me. They even refused to use John Lewin, the director in Hawaii, who was a friend and avid supporter of the Clintons. John wasn't just a public health expert; he was an energetic and astute politician who could have been important in a dozen ways. I talked about him and various others to Phil Lee, Donna Shalala's assistant secretary, and to officials in the task force. But no one had the slightest interest. It was as if the people running reform were dead set on inventing the wheel all over again.

That mentality just constantly beat on you. ASTHO had put together a major conference on health care in the twenty-first century. They had devoted a lot of thought and resources to it and had attracted a whole group of the top health professionals in the country to give papers and lead panels. But Magaziner, Shalala, and the others didn't want to be involved in any way. They didn't want to know anything about it.

But it might have been the partisanship that was the hardest thing for me to deal with. For three years the Bush administration had been developing health reform legislation. Louis Sullivan had asked me to participate in that, and I had been on the rural health advisory committee and on the infant mortality task force headed by Lawton Chiles, then senator from Florida. I was also involved with the group looking at insurance coverage in large corporations. These groups, mine and the others, had gone a long way toward developing first-rate plans, drawing on some of the most knowledgeable people available, including individuals from business and the health coverage industry.

These plans weren't secret. On the contrary, but they had absolutely no place in what was now going on. I began drawing attention to them, talking about them and asking why didn't we start from there, even if there were things we might not agree with. And why didn't we invite some of those people in, from the AMA, the Blues, the major corporation health managers, even someone like Gail Wilensky herself? But the attitude was simply, We don't want anything from the Republicans. I don't know exactly where that decision originated, but it was reflected right through the health care reform organization.

I'm as Democrat as the next person, but willfully to throw that level of work down the sinkhole I found incomprehensible. And I'm not even talking politically, from the standpoint of getting bipartisan backing for what we needed to do and not alienating major elements of the health care community that had contributed to those plans. If you really want to solve complex health and social problems like these, you look to who has answers, not to what their party is. I was so frustrated by all this at first that I felt disoriented. I wasn't sure where I fitted in exactly. Those committees under Bush had been a whole lot easier to work with. You got the sense they were out there trying to find answers, not spending their time excluding Democrats.

At some point after I understood that none of my suggestions or recommendations was going to get anywhere, I took stock and made up my mind just to buckle down. I think I decided that I wasn't going to keep upsetting myself, that there are times in life when you just have to be a good soldier and keep your mouth shut. Besides, despite my misgivings, the fact was that the committees were addressing glaring problems. We all believed that every American had to have health coverage. Health costs did have to be contained, or else we'd end up bankrupting ourselves. So I definitely felt that good was going to come of it, which turned out to be right. At the end of the day many good things did come of it.

So I listened and participated and made my suggestions gently. When I really didn't like something or other, I mainly shook my head and looked out the window. But there were one or two items that pushed me beyond my limits, that I tried hard to keep from going forward. One of those, the universal immunization bill, was outside health care reform per se. But it was important. Not just for what it was, but because it was the first health proposal the Clinton administration was pushing, so it had a precedent-setting importance too. On this one I found myself listening to people who had never in their lives been on the inside of a health department, had never seen an immunization, and probably never would see one. So of course it just had to come out entirely wrong.

Basically the administration wanted to make sure every child in the country was fully vaccinated by age two. To do that, they were proposing that the federal government buy, store, and distribute the vaccine stock. Philosophically that might have sounded like a noble idea. But the people who were advising on this were not people who knew anything about the actual system already in place. They had no clue how disruptive their proposal was going to be in practice, or why, or what would have been better.

The main fact they ignored was that the cost and availability of vaccines weren't the problem. In the eighties and early nineties Dale Bumpers and others had been successful at getting federal money for states to buy vaccines. Even before that the government's 317 Program had funded state vaccine purchases as long as the states agreed to provide free vaccinations. Medicaid also paid for vaccinations for children who qualified.

The administration bill would have had the federal government itself providing all the vaccines and storing them, which you have to be extremely careful about. This would have required special storage and handling facilities, which weren't yet available. It would have created a whole new paperwork burden. As a result, it would have disrupted the current system without being ready to substitute for it.

That was number one. More important was that the states already had all the free vaccine stock they could use. None of them had ever once run out. The problem wasn't the stock. It was administering vaccinations to the kids and making sure that data systems were in place so you had records on who had gotten what and when they needed to get their follow-ups. To increase their immunization rates, states needed money for nurses and outreach programs and computerized tracking systems. They needed infrastructure; they didn't need the government taking over vaccines.

The other big problem this bill didn't address was research costs. Drug company markups on existing vaccines helped pay for their research on new vaccines, which was of course a vexed question anyway in the way drugs are priced. But nothing in this bill addressed that question, which left a lot of people fearful that if the government bought all the vaccine at prices it set, it might upend private research efforts.

I had been involved in vaccination problems ever since the seventies, when Betty Bumpers used to make me and the other professors get out on the street corners with our syringes. After I became health director, she and Rosalynn Carter conducted a nationwide immunization campaign, and I spent a couple of days flying all over Arkansas, showing them what we were doing. Betty Bumpers had motivated her husband on this subject, and he was the acknowledged expert in the Senate. But the administration hadn't consulted him either.

I don't know how Dale Bumpers might have tried to get himself heard on this. But if he did, he wasn't listened to, and he ended up opposing this bill. The health directors, the ones on the front lines of the statewide immunization programs, also hadn't been consulted and were extremely unhappy. I set up a telephone conference with all of them to hear their objections and recommendations.

Had this been Arkansas, I would have marched over to the governor's mansion to discuss it. Of course in Washington it doesn't work that way. I thought I could probably get to see Clinton on this if I really exerted myself. But that would have considerably upset Secretary Shalala as well as those at the White House who controlled access. Instead I went through channels. I had a meeting with Assistant Secretary of HHS Phil Lee and another with Dr. D. A. Henderson of Johns Hopkins, who had been appointed to head the proposed government program. Dr. Henderson was famous for overseeing the eradication of smallpox in India. But smallpox was a one-inoculation affair, which made completely different demands on a vaccination system from those we were facing, so his experience didn't leave Dr. Henderson well prepared in this area. My meetings with Lee, then with Henderson and his top people were cordial enough. But either they weren't listening, or the administration had already made up its mind to plow ahead regardless, which I assumed was the case.

———

All this was going on before I actually became surgeon general, so I was getting a kind of foretaste of the truth that in Washington it's not just your enemies you have to watch out for. But that was only making me look forward to my confirmation even more. At least once that was over, I'd be able to get settled in and start defining my own role. As it was, not only was I following other people's agendas up here, but I was still serving as health director in Arkansas, where we had just finished seeing our new budget through the session. I had no illusions that the confirmation was going to be easy—I had too many enemies on the far right to just be ushered through—but I was really eager to have the debate done and get it behind me.

Chapter 20

Dancing with the Bear

❧❦❧

Before the confirmation hearings opened in July, Betty Bumpers was showing me around and having me meet people. One day we were up in the Senate dining room for lunch. While we were waiting for a table, senators and their guests were coming by, and Betty was stopping some of them so she could introduce me. "There's Nickles," she said. We knew Don Nickles, the conservative antiabortion Republican from Oklahoma, was going to be one of the important opposition people, and she wanted us at least to be able to say hello. "Senator," Betty said as he came by, "I want you to meet Dr. Elders."

Nickles looked away. "I don't think I need to meet Dr. Elders," he said.

Nickles aside, almost all the senators I started visiting with were extremely courteous, including those who opposed my nomination, like Orrin Hatch. Orrin Hatch might strongly disagree with me. "On that point," he'd say, "we just have to put a pin in that and differ." But he was never anything except polite. If he had been from the South, I would have called him a southern gentleman.

Other Republicans, like Alan Simpson, might not have been happy with all my positions, but were still friendly. "Well, Dr. Elders," Simpson said, "I don't agree with some of the things you're talking about, like condoms in schools. But I do think there's a problem. And maybe you can handle some problems that others of us haven't had the experience to deal with. You don't have to worry about my vote."

Mark Hatfield from Oregon showed me his collection of Lincoln books and memorabilia that are kind of the centerpiece of his office. He told me his daughter and son-in-law had just gotten their M.D.'s from the Oregon Health Science University, where I had given the commencement speech a month earlier. Apparently they had told him he was supposed to do everything he could for me. The university chancellor had too, and Hatfield said he wasn't going to disappoint any of them. If there was anything I needed, I should just call him.

I did end up calling him, which I'm sure neither of us expected. The committee hearing began on July 23, which unfortunately was the day of Vincent Foster's funeral in Little Rock. Arkansas's senators, Bumpers and David Pryor, flew down to be there, which meant I was left with no one to introduce me formally to the committee. When I told the HHS legislative people I was going to ask Hatfield, they said, "He won't do that. He's a Republican!" But I called anyway. "Senator, this is Joycelyn Elders," I said. "You told me if I ever needed you, to call. Well, I hoped I wouldn't have to, but I need you now." Then I asked if he'd introduce me.

"Dr. Elders," he said, "that's not a problem at all. I'll be happy to do that. What time do I need to be there?"

Arlen Specter was another Republican who reached out. No one was kinder to me than he was, from the moment I walked in his office and he introduced me around by telling his staff, "This is going to be our next surgeon general." But even while we were all smiling at each other I was having a hard time over what Specter had done during the Clarence Thomas/Anita Hill episode.

Specter had really stuck in my mind from the way he went after Anita Hill then. I think the reason I had focused on him even more than the others on that committee was that Specter had done so many positive things for women over a long number of years. He had also been evenhanded and open on racial issues right from the start, really a very strong history of fairness. If some old mossback had attacked Hill like that, you wouldn't mind so much because you'd expect it. But when Specter did, it was painful, especially since that confirmation was so horribly destructive to black Americans and so demeaning in particular to black women.

Specter had used all his DA skills to try to bring Anita Hill down. But if God had asked me who was telling the truth and who was lying, I would have told Him that Clarence Thomas was the liar. Hill had no reason not to be telling the truth. I didn't know Thomas, but I knew a lot of Thomases. Treating her that way would not in the least have been out of character for him, more in character than out. Nor was there anything surprising about her not reporting him at the time or his not hindering her career after she rejected him. When it comes to jobs and careers, black Americans will almost never do anything to hurt each other. They might have a fistfight in the hallway, but seldom will you hear of one black person going after another black person that way. Historically jobs have just been too hard to get, so there's a cultural inhibition against it.

I didn't feel deeply upset that Anita Hill was harassed. As far as I'm concerned, if somebody says something nasty to me, even though my job's important, I feel up to putting him in his place. Anita Hill was grown-up and capable. But that Republican committee attack on her was a spectacle, a group of powerful white males trying to destroy an innocent black woman to achieve a political goal. And using a black man to do it. I am really hostile about that, still today, sitting in my house, thinking about it at my kitchen table. I'm not hostile about a lot of things, but I'm hostile about that. I can never forgive Clarence Thomas for allowing himself to be used that way.

But my harshest feelings are reserved for the sight of someone like Thomas taking Thurgood Marshall's place. In my opinion, Thomas is a man who has sold out his black people in order to be accepted by the white establishment. Having him on the Supreme Court is the worst thing that has happened to African

Americans in recent memory. George Bush, you know, did good things for a lot of black people. His administration established a three-hundred-million-dollar fund to help save and develop the historically black colleges. The Bush family personally gave major donations to Morehouse, and Mrs. Bush sat on their board. But George Bush also made us pay dues. That nomination was the dues, and as far as I'm concerned, the price was too high.

Putting a Clarence Thomas up to replace an individual of Thurgood Marshall's stature just violated everything I believe in. It made me know that my government would stick a knife through my heart and tell me it was good for me. I still can't get over it. And Arlen Specter, despite all his history as a moderate and decent legislator, had lent himself to that.

That's why for me getting to know Arlen Specter was complicated. I was grateful for his support. I liked him personally, and I respected his record, but then there was that image of him badgering away at Anita Hill. If that wasn't tangled enough, the doctor in me got involved too. When I met Specter, he was just recovering from brain cancer surgery. His head was shaven, and the scars were still prominent. Maybe somebody else can be mad at a person who has just gone through what he did, but I have a hard time with it.

———

My hearing in front of the Labor and Human Resources Committee had been delayed. It was first scheduled for July 16, but the Republicans asked for a postponement, during which conservative newspapers let fly with a barrage of attacks. A lot of that was "Dr. Elders is a hate-filled bigot"–type comments from people like Phyllis Schlafly or that my real secret agenda was to "liberate children from traditional sexual morality." That was from the Washington *Times,* but it was a common theme. One of the battle cries was that I was a "condom queen," whatever that was supposed to mean. I told them that if I could get every teenager who engaged in sex to use a condom, I'd gladly wear a crown of condoms on my head. The Christian right flooded committee members with so many letters it almost felt like I was back in Little Rock.

When the hearing did start a week later, the Republicans tried another last-minute delaying tactic. Ted Kennedy, who chaired the committee, was buzzing with anger. "I'm not going to be part of an effort to put this over for another day or for another week," he told Indiana Senator Dan Coats, the opposition leader on the committee, "to permit scurrilous accusations to be made against this nominee without an opportunity for her to respond."

Kennedy wouldn't put up with it. He forced the hearing to go through that day, although there was enough incriminating and accusing to have taken up two or three more sessions if they had wanted. Oliver and Chester were in the gallery through it all. I was just glad my mother wasn't there to hear.

The vote was 14 to 3, but afterward the committee submitted 230 written questions for me to answer. A few were probably legitimate, even though the FBI had done a complete background investigation that pretty much answered everything but the ideological ones. But most of those questions had only one purpose: to manufacture another opportunity for delay before the confirmation went to the full Senate. The Republicans were hoping that if they had time, they could build up sufficient criticism so it would look like I was being overwhelmed. You could never tell what might happen. If they made it hard enough, maybe Clinton would pull the plug. Zoe Baird and Lani Guinier weren't that far back. Maybe I'd get so upset I'd pull the plug myself.

Kennedy had enough clout to get the full Senate floor debate scheduled for August 4 and 5. But he didn't have enough to bring it to a vote, so in the end he had to agree to another month's delay. I don't know that much actually happened during that time, except that it was a bonanza for Pat Robertson and Jerry Falwell and the other right-to-life groups, several of which looked like they were doing their lobbying out of Don Nickles's office. They pushed for that postponement because they were raising millions of dollars a week through letters pleading for money so they could keep this horrible person from becoming surgeon general. I was the best fund-raising item these religious economists had had in a long time.

I'm writing this now during the 1996 primaries, where the political strength of the Christian Coalition is a regular item of commentary. It wasn't too much less in the fall of 1993, when I was confirmed. Already back then politicians were concerned about alienating religious voters. It's possible that given the deep antagonism the Christian right felt toward my nomination, a sizable number of senators would have been concerned enough to vote against me. But I was fortunate to have my own religious supporters, the first of whom, of course, was Chester.

My involvement with the Methodists has gone back as far as I have any memory, back to before I was Sunday school secretary at our church in Schaal when I was ten. The United Methodist Women gave me my scholarship to Philander Smith, which was a church college that had been founded as a seminary. I have always been a regular churchgoer, and after Chester had come to Little Rock, I got more seriously involved. I gave talks all over the country to Methodist congregations and board meetings and was invited to be the keynote speaker at the annual Global Gathering in March before my confirmation hearings. I had done so much speaking for Methodist causes that the previous fall they had even made me layperson of the year.

The result was that at the same time the legislators were getting deluged by the Christian Coalition, they were also getting an earful from the Methodists. Chester had recently been made the church's district superintendent in South Arkansas, and I think he must have been in touch with every Methodist bishop in the country and every church organization. There was a whole lot of letter writing and telephoning going on, including from pastors of members of Congress. Organizations of Presbyterians, Jews, Church of Christ, Unitarians, and even Catholics were endorsing me too, along with groups like the YWCA and the National Council of Churches, so the religious feeling wasn't all in one direction by any means. Methodists tend not to be as loud as the Robertsons and Falwells. But they're organized, there are a lot of them, and they do have strong convictions.

After a lot of rancor, typified by the face-off between Kennedy and McCain, the Senate debate finally ended on September 7. I was confirmed by a healthy bipartisan vote, but I don't think anybody believed the opposition had run out of steam. The old Methodist bishop of Little Rock, Kenneth Hicks, used to say that when you're dancing with a bear, you can't get tired and just sit down. You have to wait for the bear to get tired, and then you can sit down. Given the level of emotion, I wasn't expecting to be doing much sitting.

In a way all the controversy might have been a little surprising. Everett Koop and Toni Novello had both called for sex education and advocated the use of condoms. It's true, I was prochoice in addition, but nobody would have expected Bill Clinton's nominee to be antichoice. What it really came down to, I think, was that I was so extremely visible. I was high-profile. I got people's attention, and the far right knew it. That made me a real threat to what they were about.

———

Oliver would have liked to carry Leona with us when we moved to Washington, but we both knew we'd have to get ourselves set up first. During the confirmation we had been living mostly in the Holiday Inn; now we had to make arrangements to move our things and get settled into the surgeon general's residence. Only after that could we start looking for someone to help out.

That meant putting Leona in a nursing home in Little Rock while we were going through the move. Once we were organized and everything was running smoothly, we were planning to bring her up. But we never got to do that. By the time we were in the new house she had become too weak to move. Not long afterward she developed pneumonia, and at the beginning of December she succumbed to it. Leona was ninety or ninety-one when she passed, we weren't absolutely sure. She had been one of the very finest people I ever knew, the most charitable and giving of herself. In a way it was fitting that her heart was the last thing about her to give out.

————

Meanwhile I was finding it almost as hard to set up my office as to get my household shipped in from Arkansas. Actually the surgeon general has two offices, a modest one in the Health and Human Services building and a large suite on the eighteenth floor of the Federal Building in Rockville, Maryland, where the Commissioned Corps has its administrative staff. When I went out to Rockville, the office there looked like a junk bin. It was huge, with a kitchen, a living room, a conference room, an assistant's office, and secretarial bays, and the whole place had furniture scattered around and holes in the ceiling tiles. I was told that Toni Novello had almost never used it.

The downtown office was just one room and would have been much more comfortable except that if you didn't count the broken-down desk and rickety chair, it was completely empty. There wasn't a bookcase or a lamp or a filing cabinet, or any files either. You would have thought I was the first surgeon general and there hadn't been any others. If you wanted to look at Luther Terry's famous surgeon general's report on smoking, for instance, you'd need to get it brought over from the Library of Congress or somewhere. The whole place was stripped bare. I was grateful when Everett Koop stopped by with a couple of boxes of stationery he had saved from his tenure. If he had thought to bring some pens and pencils, I could have used those too.

I was not absolutely positive the reception I was getting in Secretary Shalala's office was a lot more hospitable. Dr. Lee, the assistant secretary, was a man I already knew I could work with. He had previously been vice-president at the University of San Francisco Medical School and he had a no-nonsense, straightforward manner. But I thought my interactions with Donna Shalala might have been a little bit schizophrenic. My first exposure to that was back in January during the inauguration. Shalala had seemed very friendly and had invited me to meet with her the next morning in her office. But when I got there, a secretary said she was too busy to see me; if I needed something, I should call her later.

That kind of business started repeating itself when I finally moved in. Shalala would ask me to be with her for some speech or event, but when I'd show up at her office, she would seem surprised and annoyed that I was there. It was a strange way to act, to say the least. I assumed she knew that I had initially talked to Clinton about the secretary's job, and for all I know I might actually have been in contention at one point. I had gotten that call from Louis Sullivan, so he must have heard it from somewhere. But that was a million years back, and it wasn't credible that she'd have any insecurity about such a thing. Yet she seemed to go out of her way. "I didn't pick Dr. Elders," she'd make a point of telling people. "I hired Oliver Elders, but I didn't hire Joycelyn Elders." There wasn't exactly an open antagonism there, but I think most people felt that something was going on.

Actually, in the end Oliver's job as executive director of the President's Council on Sports and Physical Fitness never did come through. We were in the middle of working out the details when it was decided that the council would be one of my responsibilities as deputy assistant secretary. That meant Oliver couldn't be director, because he'd be working for me. I didn't push it too hard, although from where I was sitting, it looked like that office could have just as easily been moved someplace else on the organizational chart. Instead Oliver got a position at the Department of Education as special assistant to the secretary. Just on general principles I always thought it was a waste to spend energy going around getting things officially changed, unless somebody's life or health might have depended on it. But that Council on Sports and Physical Fitness was one thing I probably should have worked to get done.

One reason I didn't might have been that right from the start I was moving fast. Dr. Lee was talking about how his three deputies would be running the department's programs with him, but for me, at least, it didn't necessarily work out that way. That wasn't Dr. Lee's fault. I just wasn't there enough. The others were in the office, but I tended to be out traveling— giving speeches, meeting people, and making appearances in different corners of the country.

In the fifteen months I was surgeon general I gave 302 speeches. When I do the math, it's a wonder I can still distinguish even a few of them. But some were memorable, like the extemporaneous commencement address I gave at Harvard after my briefcase with my speech and good shoes in it had inexplicably disappeared during lunch at the Faculty Club. That was almost as challenging as an appearance I once made along with some other dignitaries where they put Texas Governor Ann Richards's speech up on the TelePrompTer instead of mine. It took me a minute or two to get my bearings on that one, and in the meantime I was reading Ann's words. Unless they all were just being polite, neither she nor anyone else seemed to notice.

Given the moment, many of my speeches had to do with health care reform. On this subject I picked what I personally wanted to talk about and push. I talked about universal health coverage not just as a necessity but as a right. Historically, I told my audiences, major social legislation comes along every thirty years. Workers' compensation began in 1902, Social Security during the thirties, then Medicare and Medicaid in the sixties. Every thirty-year generation sees an enlargement of understanding about what kind of minimum safety net the community should provide for its members. Now the right of everyone to see a doctor was due.

But it bothered me that just about the whole public debate was about how to manage acute care or hospital care—what I called sick care. The fact is, the country already has a very good sick care system, the best in the world. What we don't have is a health care system, one that's oriented to keeping people healthy instead of treating them when they're sick. That is the key to massively raising the health standards of Americans and, not at all incidentally, to dramatically lowering the health bill.

That was my theme: moving from sick care to health care. We need to have everyone covered. But along with that what we really want is to find ways to keep them healthy. I grasped hold of this preventive approach to health—actually I had been grasping on to it for years—and I went out to sell it.

In my speeches I used the example of immunization: huge health benefits and fourteen dollars saved for every dollar spent. I told my audiences how much cheaper and more effective it was to train bus drivers to make sure diabetic children get their snacks than to have doctors treat their crises. Our studies had shown that in rural America 35 percent of families did not have the transportation to get to a doctor conveniently. How much cheaper it was to provide transportation for checkups than to wait for the crisis that requires emergency service. In Maryland, I told them, the highest incidence of blindness was to be found within a mile radius of the Johns Hopkins Eye Institute. The sufferers were usually over sixty-five, which meant they had Medicare. But most were simply unaware of the services available. Here, as so often elsewhere, education was far and away the cheapest and most effective treatment.

I outlined for my audiences the elements of a preventive health care system. Providing medical services where people live, work, and go to school. Training more primary care doctors. Increasing incentives for doctors to practice in underserved areas. Training more minority doctors and nurses. Providing outreach like transportation, visiting care providers, translation services, community education and mobilization. Emphasizing immunizations, prenatal checkups, screenings, and physicals. What we needed to do, I said, is invest in these approaches and link them together so that we could provide an integrated, comprehensive preventive health care service. We needed to make sure people had financial access, physical access, and cultural access.

But first, middle, and last, we needed education. Despite everything, we still have a largely health-illiterate society. People have to be taught what services are available and how to use them. They have to be educated to keep themselves healthy, not in some haphazard, catch-as-catch-can way, but through thorough, comprehensive health education from kindergarten through graduation, so that young people will develop a health foundation early in life that they can build on the rest of their lives. No number of doctors can do for people's health what people can do for themselves. But if they are going to take care of themselves, they have to know how. They have to be made aware. And that was exactly how I saw my role as surgeon general. I was in office to make them aware.

Right from the start speaking invitations flowed in, and I accepted as many as I could. Very quickly speeches started bunching up, one after another. My speech writers were often bent out of shape because they'd send speeches over to the White House for vetting and would get them back torn down and reoriented. I told them, "Don't worry about what they do to those speeches over there. I'm not giving those speeches anyway." I counted on my writers to give me background and context and data, but I had never in my life just read off a speech someone else wrote down for me. So there hardly seemed much point in their fighting over the wording of some sentence I probably wasn't going to use anyway.

Often as not I didn't even know what speech had been sent to the White House for them to look at. I was on the road speaking half the time, and the other half I was speaking in Washington. It was a lot of speeches. I knew that not everything I said was completely in line with the administration's positions. I personally didn't believe that the people who were guiding health care reform had any particular understanding of the base rock necessity of preventive health anyway.

I also didn't take well to heavy-handed attempts to control my schedule. At one point I signed on to give a talk at the annual convention of the National Lesbian and Gay Journalists Association, which had been cofounded by the HHS deputy secretary for public affairs, Victor Zonana. Then I noticed it had been taken off my calendar. Somebody in the secretary's office apparently thought the forum was too sensitive. That was exactly the kind of thing I didn't have any time for. I put it back on and went anyway.

I guess there were some disadvantages to running around as much as I was, the main one being that I wasn't spending any time taking care of my political flanks. Often I wasn't current with everything going on behind the scenes at HHS, and I practically never saw anybody at all from the White House. My impression was that President Clinton figured I could take care of myself, which was just fine with me. Shalala, I knew, was not a friend, and I never went out of my way to cultivate allies who might help compensate for that. Somehow that just didn't seem like the kind of thing I ought to be spending my time doing. My chief of staff, Carol Roddy, suggested a number of times that I go over and meet Leon Panetta, especially after some flap or other. But I never did. "I don't have anything to tell him," I said, "so what would I see him for?" But she might have known something I didn't. The first time I ever did talk to Panetta was a year later, when he called to demand my resignation.

———

I know that particular possibility never occurred to me as December began rolling toward Christmas. It was hard to believe I had only been in office for a little over three months. I had barely had time to catch my breath.

On December 7 I gave a talk at the National Press Club. I don't remember that there was anything especially controversial in it. But in the question and answer session afterward, a reporter asked if I thought legalizing drugs would lower the crime rate. I said, "Yes, I do feel that we would markedly reduce our crime rate if drugs were legalized." Then I said, "But I don't know the consequences. Perhaps it's something that ought to be studied."

Now, I don't know that there's much controversial about that either. I wasn't advocating legalization, like William F. Buckley was, for instance. And there isn't a criminologist in the country who doesn't think the crime rate would drop the day after drugs were legalized or decriminalized. All I had said was that maybe the question should be studied.

But that was enough; it was more than enough. The next day explosions were lighting off everywhere you looked. It felt like a walking barrage from World War I. Most of the attacks accused me of leading the charge for legalization. When you put this together with my position on making condoms available and my prochoice stance, it was enough to send my critics blasting into orbit. There was so much noise that President Clinton felt he had to announce that even studying the legalization of drugs was not in any way the policy of his administration.

———

Eight days later Victor Zonana, the deputy secretary, came into my office looking troubled. "Dr. Elders," he said, "we just picked up this AP report. It says there's a warrant out for the arrest of a Kevin Elders, age twenty-eight, in Little Rock. On a drug charge."

Chapter 21

A Bend in the Road

Kevin and drugs was not something Oliver or I had thought about for three or four years now. It wasn't something either of us wanted to think about ever again. Kevin was a grown man, doing well, as kind and caring as he had always been, with his addictions behind him, so far as we could see. He came to visit us sometimes, and sometimes we went over to his place. Since those bad old days I had never seen him so much as take a drink except once. He and Oliver were watching a basketball game or something and Kevin went into the icebox and came out with a beer. My stomach fell about two feet. "Kevin!" I said. I was upset. "I know you're twenty-eight years old and can decide for yourself. But you *know* I remember those problems. Do you need to start going back to your AA meetings?"

"No, no, Mom," he said. "What are you talking about?" And that was the only time.

The minute after I saw that AP story I was on the line to Little Rock. Kevin was home; he hadn't been arrested. That was a relief all by itself. When I told him, he said he didn't know anything about it. This was the first he had heard of any warrant. As soon as I got off with Kevin, I called our lawyer, to have him find out what was going on. Awhile later he called back. Yes, he said, it was true. An arrest warrant for Kevin had been issued; the police just hadn't picked him up yet. According to the charge, Kevin had sold someone an eighth of an ounce of cocaine. Supposedly that had happened the previous summer, on July 29. No, he didn't have any idea why they had waited till now to put out the warrant.

The only reason Oliver and I weren't desperate that night was that Kevin was saying he hadn't done it. It must be some kind of fabrication or mix-up. So we latched on to that and tried to act like it was nothing to worry about. We had been down this road before, and we weren't eager to go back. If Kevin was saying he hadn't done anything, maybe he hadn't. Besides, it was very peculiar that right after I had mentioned legalizing drugs, all of a sudden my son would get picked up on a drug charge.

The next day Kevin went down to the police station with the lawyer and turned himself in. Bond was set at $250, which didn't exactly sound like some kind of major crime had been committed. So that helped Oliver and me stay in containment mode. We were going to find out what was up soon enough. Until then we were just not going to worry about it.

Of course there was no way of ignoring it either. By now Kevin's arrest was splattered across every front page in the country. There hadn't even been time for the shouting about legalization to die down yet. So to have this happen now was like throwing fresh meat to sharks. The kinder ones were suggesting that Kevin was the reason I was pushing legalization in the first place. Not that I was pushing it, but that didn't matter. The unkinder ones were saying that here I was supposed to be the nation's doctor and I couldn't even care for my own children.

One comforting voice was Bill Clinton's. A day after the news hit he called to talk. He was very sorry to hear about Kevin, he said. He understood about these things himself, all too well, because of the problems his brother, Roger, had had. It was tough. He knew Oliver and I would find a way to bear up, and he wanted us to know that his thoughts and Hillary's were with us.

It was good talking with Clinton, especially since the clamor over what had happened was only getting worse. I had to figure out very quickly how to respond to it because I could not even get out the front door of my house in the morning or my office at night the phone was so busy with people calling to ask me about my son. And I don't mean calling to say, "Oh, Dr. Elders, I'm so sorry to hear, and could you tell me about it?" At meetings where I was speaking people would stand up and say, "Well, you know, you're out here talking to other people about things while you should have been at home taking care of your son. What do you have to say about that?" It got very harsh.

Well, I thought about my answer. I thought about how I felt. And the way I felt was that Kevin is my child and I'm his mother. I don't always approve of everything my children do. But that doesn't make me any less their mother. I always have been, and I always will be. That was how I felt about Kevin, which was exactly the way I had always felt about both him and Eric. Neither the surgeon general's job nor any other job could make the slightest difference in that.

Meanwhile I coped the way I have always coped, by speeding up. I've been lucky in my life that I've always had more work to do than I have time for. When something happens that threatens to overwhelm me, I get real busy. There's never not been one more job to do or one more patient to see, which keeps me from getting preoccupied. I hadn't faced many situations worse than this with Kevin, but every time I felt I couldn't stand it any longer, I'd find something else that needed doing. I consumed myself with work.

It was worse for Oliver, I think, much worse. I get hyper; he broods. He sits there and thinks about it and stews over it. He turns it around again and again. He's tough, but his shell is more brittle than mine. He will weather it, but his weathering doesn't diminish the hurt. Oliver was a teacher and a coach all his life. He was a model for young men that practically the whole state looked up to. All I had to do was think about how it was that I had failed my son.

At first we didn't know the details. After Kevin posted bond, he went back to work every day, and it was hard to talk on the phone. We had planned to go back home for Christmas, but instead we had Kevin come up and spend it in Washington. But even face-to-face it was hard to talk. We were still doing our best to delude ourselves into thinking that maybe there really wasn't a problem. But at the same time we were telling him, "You know, if you need treatment, you've got to go and get it." Kevin himself was saying nothing. He wasn't saying, "Yes, I need treatment," or, "No, I don't need it." He mostly just listened. Then every once in a while he'd say he didn't want to talk about it.

Maybe that should have raised our suspicions higher. Sitting here and talking about it now, two years later, I can scarcely believe it didn't. Especially since we were not newcomers. But still, when it's your child, you naturally crave that state of denial, so badly do you want it not to be.

The trial was in July 1994, six months later. By then we knew a lot of the facts. We knew that one of Kevin's friends, Calvin Walraven, had been after Kevin to get some cocaine for him. He had started asking him at the beginning of July 1993. Then, when Kevin kept refusing, he got more and more insistent.

I knew Calvin; at least I had met him. A couple of times Kevin had brought him over to the house, a white boy Kevin's age who looked down on his luck. Another stray. Kevin was always picking up strays. Somewhere in those six months Kevin admitted to us that he and Calvin did drugs together, not often but sometimes. He told us that he had not stopped after that last treatment program he had been through down near Grambling. He told us he was still an addict.

According to Kevin, he had fended off Calvin's pleas for almost a month, with Calvin calling him numerous times every day. Finally Calvin told him that if Kevin didn't do it, he was going to go public about Kevin's addiction. That was on July 28. My nomination was scheduled to go before the full Senate seven days later. Kevin feared what might happen, he told us; his mind was clouded. He decided to go ahead and get the drugs.

Kevin's trial was set for July 18, 1994. A few days before it started a call came into my office from a friend of mine in Little

Rock who was a psychiatrist. She told me she was calling about Kevin's case. Calvin Walraven had been her patient for some time, she said. In fact he was in her office with her at the moment. He had given her permission to call. There were things he wanted to tell me that she thought might exonerate Kevin. Would I get on the phone with him?

When Calvin came on the line, he was obviously in distress. His voice was hoarse and quavering. He was sorry, he said. He was so very sorry. The police had made him do it; they had paid him and threatened him. They were after Kevin because of me. Was there some way I could please get him out of testifying, because he didn't want to do it? He was so sorry.

When he got off, my friend told me that Calvin was staying in a psychiatric facility under medication. He had a long history of mental problems and drug addiction. He was suffering acutely.

Three days before the trial Kevin was offered a deal by the prosecutor. If he pled guilty to a lesser charge of delivering drugs, the prosecutor would recommend a shorter sentence than what he would get for selling. Kevin absolutely refused. Yes, he said, he was an addict. But he had been forced into doing this. Never in his life had he been a dealer.

At the trial Calvin was the main witness. He came in under some kind of heavy sedation, his pupils dilated and his eyes glazed. On the stand he told a story of trying to get Kevin to buy drugs for him for weeks, calling him at least once a day, sometimes more. When Kevin agreed, he had arranged a place and time to meet, but he didn't come alone. An undercover police officer was in his car, and another was hiding out nearby, watching.

Our lawyer argued entrapment, that Kevin wasn't a dealer and that the police used his friend to get him to do something he wouldn't otherwise have done. But in his verdict the judge didn't agree. A month later he ruled that Kevin had sold 1.85 grams of cocaine. In Arkansas the minimum sentence for that was ten years in prison. In fact during its previous session the Arkansas legislature had changed that mandatory sentence to probation, but the change hadn't gone into effect until August 13, two weeks after Kevin had committed his offense. So Kevin was sentenced to ten years in jail. Calvin wasn't there to hear the verdict. A week after the trial he shot himself to death in a motel room in Hot Springs. I remembered his eyes after he had testified when he had come across to tell me, "I'm sorry, Mrs. Elders, I'm sorry. Please forgive me."

As soon as the trial was over, Kevin went into intensive treatment, first at a center in Little Rock, then at a program in Fort Smith. He was in treatment when the verdict came down and when we started our appeals. The appeals were mainly based on a piece of evidence that had not come out at the trial. Although the prosecution is supposed to make all the evidence available to the defense, the state attorney had not revealed that Calvin had been a paid police informant. It could be that the prosecutor hadn't known; the police might have kept the information from him. Police records showed that they had paid Calvin $155 for Kevin's arrest. At the trial they had presented him as someone who volunteered his information only because he was Kevin's friend and wanted to get him off drugs.

When I talked to a friend of mine who is a federal judge about appealing, he said, "Joycelyn, you will not win that. If you want to make the appeal for Kevin, to let him know you're behind him, fine. But don't expect to win; the judicial climate won't allow it. So think hard before you throw all your money into following the first one up. You're not going to do anything here but lose."

Well, we did lose the first one. And we lost the second. After that they were ready to take Kevin into prison, and even though another appeal was coming up, we all felt that Kevin should begin doing his time. On August 7, 1995, he went in. This was after I had already been out of office for almost a year. Taking Kevin down to the court and watching him go off isn't something that's easy to describe. We were praying that he would somehow find a way to turn what was happening into something positive.

It might sound strange to say, but I have mixed feelings about everything that's gone on with Kevin. I'm not a suspicious person by nature, and I've tried not to think this, but I can't help wondering about the coincidences. The police went after Calvin Walraven to get Kevin at the beginning of July, just when I was formally nominated. They arrested Kevin five months later, right after my drug legalization remark. Maybe there are innocent reasons for that, I don't know. But I do know the climate in Arkansas, where Bill Clinton's political enemies have made it their business never to let him rest from allegations and embarrassments. I will probably go down to my grave not knowing if my family suffered too from this politics of hatred that has been waged against the President.

But I say my feelings are mixed. Because for all the misery we've gone through, what happened with Kevin is a blessing. A year after he was convicted, before he went into prison, Oliver and I could see the change in him. Kevin had been in treatment that entire time. He was thinking more clearly and making more sense than he had been a year back. He was no longer lying, the way drug addicts habitually do. He was no longer distant and easily distracted, giveaway signs that earlier we had just refused to see. He was beginning to have dreams and aspirations again.

Even in prison we were lucky. Kevin was sentenced to ten years, but because he was a first-time nonviolent offender he qualified for Arkansas's special Boot Camp program. Boot Camp is tough. It emphasizes physical training and military-style discipline. More than half of the prisoners wash out. Kevin didn't. He stuck it out. For the three months he was there Oliver and I used to drive up and park off a ways where we could see Kevin from a distance through the fencing and where he could see us.

Boot Camp goes for three months, and afterward graduates are allowed out on probation. As I write this, Kevin is living at home with us. Chester sometimes accuses me. He says that Mama only had an eighth-grade education while I've got more years of school than a person can easily count. But for all that difference, he doesn't think that in some respects I got the slightest bit farther than Mama. When it comes to faith, I don't know a thing more than what I learned from her—"primitive faith," Chester calls it. That may be so. I really do fall back on God. I believe that whatever it is, no matter how bad it might be, God would not have let it happen without a reason. We have Kevin at home now, but I feel in my heart that if his addiction had not been brought to light, eventually we would have lost him. Oliver and I would have awakened one morning to hear that he was gone. That's reason enough, I think. That helps me understand.

———

In public this was a storm I rode out. Of course, whatever I might have been feeling personally, the world was going to go on anyway. If anything, the train was gathering speed. In early 1994 the health care reform legislation was finally taking shape. As the administration's top doctor, I was involved, especially in the adolescent health portion.

The adolescent health portion had really started out as a separate bill Ted Kennedy had been drafting, something that could stand on its own as a complete piece of legislation, although inevitably it was incorporated into the big health care reform picture. The primary elements were exactly the ones I had been pushing since I was health director in Arkansas: comprehensive health education and on-site health care in schools.

I was giving speeches on these in every forum I could get to, doing everything I knew to describe the value and the necessity of these programs and give a realistic picture of them. I tried to counter the feverish sexual attacks being marshaled by the right, the same as they always had, except even more stridently now that health reform was moving toward a showdown. Health education, I said, was fundamentally necessary in developing fit, safe, responsible children. They had to be given the tools to understand and protect themselves in this dangerous world of drugs, smoking, gun violence, poor nutrition, and unsafe sex. That kind of education could not be left to chance, to parents who too often didn't know themselves or were unable to teach.

Less than 5 percent of the nation's schools had comprehensive health education programs. If you wanted to know the consequences, all you needed to do was look at the statistics. We've tried ignorance, I said. Now it's time to try education.

Ignorance is not bliss, and sex education does *not* mean teaching five-year-olds how to perform sex acts, which was the Christian right's favorite theme. Sex education means teaching youngsters self-esteem; it means teaching them to avoid abuse; it means teaching them the physiology of reproduction and the nature of disease—everything at an appropriate age. They have to know how to stay safe and healthy. They don't need instruction on the how-tos of sex. God taught all of us that.

Education is not a one-time affair; this was my favorite theme. It's not a one-semester affair. You can't get up for thirty minutes and talk about the need for safe sex and think you've done it. You have to attend to it over and over and build and build until it becomes part of people's consciousness. It takes long reaches of time to inculcate healthy habits, like persuading people not to drink and drive or not to smoke. In these kinds of things people are slow learners. It takes years of effort before it gets into their heads that if you're drinking, you don't drive. If you want to be cool, don't smoke. If you're going to have sex, use a condom. You have to teach them to play the tape out to the end, as the twelve-steppers say, so that they'll see the consequences when they think about the behavior.

If you can get less controversial than this, I'd like to know how. One op-ed piece in my favor was titled "Dr. Uncontroversial." But that wasn't how the antieducation, antichoice, condom-on-the-brain people saw it. I'd talk about health education and school-based clinics, the second major part of adolescent health. School-based clinics were mainly important for rural and poor inner-city areas, where there were large populations of needy young people whose access to doctors was limited, who didn't go, whose parents couldn't or wouldn't take them, whose families didn't have the money. School clinics would provide primary health care for youngsters—from checkups to allergy shots to asthma treatment, to counseling, to referrals to specialists. The bill set minimum requirements for schools that wanted them. They had to provide K–12 health education, and they had to be able to do referrals, including referrals to gynecologists. They did *not* have to provide condoms.

I was and am absolutely convinced that most Americans easily understand and agree with the significance and benefits of on-site primary health care. It is not the norm in the United States, where until recently everyone has been accustomed to the fee-for-service model of medical treatment. But because it hasn't been the norm doesn't mean that it's outside the mainstream. Providing medical services for poor children who don't otherwise get them isn't exactly a radical far-left notion that will destroy the nation's morality.

Yet that is precisely how the militants portrayed it. Health education meant contaminating young minds, and health services meant murdering the unborn. I am no expert on George Orwell, but I know doublespeak when I hear it. I had been hearing it a long time. I am still hearing it.

Everywhere I went, the protesters were there. They were incredibly organized. I'd go to give a speech someplace in Illinois, and they were there; in Colorado and they were there too, waving placards with photographs of aborted fetuses. They were like some kind of little terrier that's gnawing on your shoe and you can't shake it off.

Inside the auditoriums they'd get up in the question period and start making speeches. "Dr. Elders, do you know that the Bible says that life begins with . . ." It was almost always the same. Their literature tells them to get their points across in a set piece monologue before they ask a question, to get the cameras' attention and disrupt the meeting.

I'd say, "What is your question?" and they'd go back and start the speech over. At first I'd get frustrated by it. After the third time I tried to get them to ask a question I'd say, "Well, you know what? As far as I'm concerned, you're a liar. Your question's a lie, and I don't answer lies, so there's no point in you asking. Next!"

It didn't take long before I started spotting them right off and immediately demand their question. They'd say, "Do you believe in killing innocent babies?"

I'd answer, "No, I don't believe in killing innocent babies. I don't deal with people who have a love affair with the fetus but won't take care of children. I'm about taking care of babies, but I'm not about unplanned, unwanted children."

And I tried to make it very quick. I just decided I'm not going to let them do that. Not on my time.

Eventually, of course, the adolescent health segment went down in flames along with the rest of health care reform. But there's an interesting postscript to it, at least to the school-based clinics part. At the time pediatricians were opposed. They even went in and voted against it. But later, as the health industry kept revolutionizing itself, they realized that maybe it wasn't such a bad idea after all. Statistically children are a healthy group. As managed care took hold, pediatricians realized that they could be the doctors for school clinics and have all those children as part of their plan, with their nurse practitioners doing most of the work. It didn't cost very much to do that, especially since the facilities were being provided by the schools. With capitated rates, set fees per month per child, it became economically attractive. If you go to a nursing home and do capitation, you're going to sink. But if you go to an elementary school with capitation, you'll make a bundle.

The result was that the idea began spreading like wildfire. Suddenly pediatricians all thought school-based clinics were a great thing and they should be the consultant or the doctor in charge. That's an irony I muse over on occasion. If I had thought of it in economic terms, I would have gotten a clinic into every school in the country. If I had been more of an economist than a do-gooder, I could probably have had exactly what I was looking for.

———

As 1994 gathered speed, the health care reform legislation was being fought out in committees and in public. Everyone knew we had some real problems. In the first place, negative images had gotten attached to it. The secrecy that had surrounded those big committees had made the process look slightly conspiratorial. Then there was the popular picture of Magaziner at the top of this huge apparatus shifting around vast stacks of coded files to try to come up with a grand overall blueprint that integrated everything. To the opposition it was easy to make the whole thing out as the worst kind of giant government bureaucracy come to life. I personally wished that it would have been a more open process from the beginning, to defuse suspicions and allow differing views to be heard. Others outside the administration would have had a chance to buy into it. And I think we would have benefited from having a couple of more heads at the top. Actually, if the process had been inclusive instead of so intensely partisan, the organization of it might not have even mattered that much. But it wasn't.

A more serious problem was that a lot of people saw the plan as unnecessarily complicated. We all felt that we needed to make sure everybody had access to health care. But those who weren't already covered were a minority: the poor and underserved; people who were out of work or were doing part-time, low-pay jobs; children who had finished college and were in insurance limbo. And even in this group the poor and elderly had Medicaid and Medicare. We could have just concentrated on finding a way to get the uninsured minority covered. A lot of the people who had been working on this a long time were saying exactly that. Instead, to get the uninsured minority included, the plan was going to revamp the way everybody was covered.

The result was that we ended up with a complicated plan and an extremely complicated financial management system. In retrospect, if we were going to redo everybody, we probably should have gone to a single-payer system. The doctors would have been happy with that, and it would have had the virtue of relative simplicity. As it was, the plan was so complicated that it was easy to attack and hard to defend. Even after you got through explaining it, people still didn't understand. All they knew was that they were as confused as ever, and maybe you weren't too clear on it yourself, since you hadn't been able to put it plainly.

With all that, it's nevertheless true that the plan itself was pretty good. It resolved many issues that needed resolving. It would have improved medical coverage significantly and put a limit on costs. From where I'm sitting now, it seems likely that many of its elements will be passed piecemeal in one form or other in the fairly near term, with bipartisan support.

———

With universal coverage at the center of everybody's attention, I had the strong impression that we were out there trying to sell a product before people had been sold on the need for it. The fact was that most of those who were listening to the debate had coverage. They weren't completely concerned whether Joe Blow in the street had it or not. They weren't hardhearted. They'd do something about him if they could. But they weren't too eager to subject themselves to something that they didn't understand very well, that cost money, and that was so complex it might have some negative consequences as well as positive. Especially not when they weren't convinced that they themselves had all that big an investment in it.

To make matters worse, the various components of the health care industry that didn't like it had the best marketing people they could hire out campaigning against it. The administration should have had its own marketing strategy in place, the more so since we had excluded a lot of important voices, who consequently were alienated instead of invested. But it didn't, so we lost the public relations battle almost by default.

It was all over before the August recess. The chairmen—other than Kennedy—hadn't been able to move the bills out of their committees. They were struggling to get people to stay and work on them, but midterm elections were coming up, and it wasn't looking too good for the Democrats. Everyone wanted to get home and start running. When they came back in September, health care reform was deader than a doornail.

I think everybody hurt. After the immensity of the effort, not to mention the stakes, there was no way they couldn't. But I don't remember that there was any finger pointing. People hurt the way you do when you are watching your child failing. You hurt, and you start blaming yourself and feeling that if I had done this or that, maybe it wouldn't have happened. You don't blame your child. I think there was a lot of that going on. Everybody took it on himself for it to be his fault.

There was no real conclusive moment to it either, no general postmortems and no attempt to put a closure to it and restore morale by pointing out the good along with the bad. Because good did come of it. The nation became conscious of health care as it had never been, and of the need for reform. The debate itself hastened changes that are reducing costs and bringing preventive medicine into better focus. It prepared the way for legislation that will get passed. Oliver would most definitely have given a locker-room talk afterward, but maybe there wasn't time. We were already into welfare reform, and elections were bearing down hard.

———

For me personally, the defeat of health care reform was a blow. I felt we lost a lot. I was especially unhappy about the school-linked sections going down. But I saw it as a battle, not the war. For all the things I was involved in, the heart of my personal agenda was improving the health of America's adolescents. And by the fall of 1994 I thought we were well on the way to making a real difference in that area.

For more than a year now I had been working toward a conference that would set the nation's agenda for adolescent health. Many different government agencies and private organizations were taking on problems that affected teenagers: drugs, violence, STDs, unwanted pregnancy, smoking, alcohol, nutrition, exercise. What I intended to do was define and coordinate these efforts, set specific goals, and develop strategies to meet them. I wanted to take all these distinct, separate, fragmented pieces, see how they fit, and stitch them together into a quilt.

As deputy assistant secretary for adolescent health, minority health, women's health, and family planning I was perfectly situated to make this happen. As surgeon general I had the bully pulpit to draw the public's attention. Since there was no funding available for this conference, I solicited all the agencies that were involved. They responded, and excitement started to rise among people working in adolescent health. They could see this coming together, and they all wanted to be part of it. I was asking the country's acknowledged experts to contribute papers, give talks, and lead groups: academicians and fieldworkers and politicians of every stripe, four or five hundred people all told. Our intention was to pull together a nationwide plan of attack on adolescent health problems.

We had already written the white paper that was going to be the anchor and outline for the conference, with participation by leading authorities like Claire Brindis. Joy Dryfoos, and scholars from the Alan Gutmacher Institute and Robert Wood Johnson Foundation. The CDC was making a focused effort on exercise and health, ASTHO's adolescent health committee was involved; it had been working full-time on overall adolescent health for several years. The AMA was working on a book for adolescent preventive health, a kind of pamphlet for every adolescent to have as a guide to what he or she might need at different times. The president of the Robin Hood Foundation, Paul Jones, had organized a group of Wall Street and Madison Avenue social marketeers who were preparing to lay out the marketing strategy for what we were going to do and how we were going to sell this plan. The Robin Hood Foundation was also making a million dollars available to the surgeon general so that for the first time we could accurately assess the cost of teenage pregnancy to the United States.

That last one, of course, had my special attention. My seven-plus years in public health only reinforced the conclusion I first drew in Arkansas those initial few months I was director: that out-of-wedlock teenage pregnancy is *the* key factor in perpetuating the cycle of poverty. This is especially true in the black and Hispanic communities, but in the white community as well, where teenage pregnancy has also shot up wildly, with devastating social and economic results.

Education alone isn't going to solve this problem, nor will making condoms easily available. If giving away condoms were the solution, I would have been handing them out on street corners. But you make inroads with education; you create awareness. You open people's eyes to responsibility. Young men can be instructed on the obligations of fatherhood, that making a donation of sperm is not the end of it; they can also be required to contribute financially through a system of Social Security number identification.

Adolescent health services can assure teenage girls who do not want babies that family planning is available, contraceptives are available, and abortion is available if that is their choice. Frankly I have never been tremendously concerned about people with resources and education. They can be counted on to do what's right for themselves and their families. But I have always been concerned about the fourteen- or fifteen-year-old girl who has no money, who has no health coverage, who has often been raped or abused, who is afraid and does not know where to turn.

They are the ones I've directed my attention to. They are the reason, for example, that I tried to make the "morning-after pill" available. The morning-after pill is different from RU-486, the French abortifacient that is currently undergoing FDA trials. The morning-after pill is simply two tablets of one of the high-dose estrogen and progestin birth control pills like Ovral, followed by two more tablets twelve hours later; or four tablets of standard low-dose Ovral, followed by four more after twelve hours. Taken up to seventy-two hours after intercourse, these dosages prevent conception.

This is not a substitute for standard birth control. High doses like this will make you very sick to your stomach. They will nauseate you and make you vomit. A person who wanted to use birth control pills this way for contraception would very soon be turned off to sex. But if you've had an accident, or if you didn't expect to have sexual intercourse but ended up having it, then this is a way to make sure you will not get pregnant.

I wanted to have birth control pills packaged with the right dosages for use as morning-after pills and sold over the counter. Because if you feel you need a morning-after pill, you do not have time to make an appointment with a gynecologist and get a prescription filled. It's safe. I don't think the people at the FDA are worried about its safety. I was trying to get them to approve it (they eventually did, in 1996). But the drug companies did not want to package it this way because they thought that many women would stop taking the usual twenty-eight-day monthly regimen of birth control pills—especially unmarried young women who might have intercourse only sporadically or infrequently.

But as important as it was, teenage pregnancy was only one element in what I foresaw as a comprehensive treatment of adolescent health needs and how to meet them. The brightest and the best in the business were working hard on this. We were determined to put it all together and make it fly. The conference was set for April at the Ritz Carlton in Tysons Corner, Virginia, right next to Washington so members of Congress could get there. In effect, this is what I had been working toward ever since the day I left the medical school in 1987.

———

On December 1 I gave a speech at the World AIDS Day conference at the UN. Afterward during a panel discussion a psychiatrist asked me a question. The context was the necessity of breaking down taboos against talking about sex in order to counter the epidemic. Participants there were from all over the world, many from Africa, where in some places HIV rates were 50 percent, much of that through heterosexual transmission. The psychiatrist's subject was whether alternative methods of sexual release might be encouraged to inhibit the spread of the disease. "What do you think are the prospects for a discussion and promotion of masturbation?" he asked.

I might have squirmed a little at that, but not much. I told him I was a strong advocate of comprehensive health education that was age-appropriate and complete, that children had to be taught all the things they needed to know. Later on *Nightline* Ted Koppel told me it sounded as if I had been trying to avoid the question. I wasn't. I meant to answer the psychiatrist that human sexuality should be covered in health education and that masturbation was a part of human sexuality. But as I was talking to him, I thought that maybe what I had said wasn't clear enough. If I was going to say something, I wanted to say it explicitly. "In regard to masturbation," I told him, "I think that is part of human sexuality, and perhaps it should be taught." The next moment there was another question, and the panel went on to different subjects.

This was World AIDS Day, and the room was filled with media people. None of them asked about the remark. It was so innocuous that nobody seemed to notice it. The next day neither the newspapers nor the TV reported anything about it. But Donna Shalala's assistant was there, and apparently she did take notice.

A week and a half later I was having a meeting out in Rockville when a call came in from Shalala's office. She wanted to see me. I told my secretary to let her know I was in the middle of a meeting and could we make it for later? No, the answer came back, Secretary Shalala needed to see me now, and could I please be downtown at her office at ten-thirty? I had no idea what she wanted, but I thought it had to be pretty urgent to call me into Washington on the spur of the moment.

When I got there, the secretary was in her office with Dr. Lee and his chief deputy, Dr. Bouford. When I sat down, she asked whether I had said anything about masturbation during the UN conference the other week. I was wondering what she was talking about. "Yes, probably," I said.

"Did you say masturbation ought to be taught in schools?"

"Well, I don't know exactly, I think something like that." I was trying to remember precisely what I had said.

Shalala was shaking her head. "That's a real problem," she said, head shaking back and forth. "That's a real problem. I don't know what we can do about this. I don't know if we can save you this time."

What in the world is this woman talking about? I was thinking. Save me from what? Lee and Bouford were sitting there expressionless, not saying a word.

"What do you mean?" I asked.

"I just think this is too much," Shalala said. "You know, *U.S. News* is going to mention it in an article. I'm sorry it's come to this, but I've got to take it up with Panetta."

"Well." I got up to leave. "Thanks for telling me."

"Where are you going to be?" she asked.

"I'll be back out at Rockville," I said.

On the drive back out I was fuming. Why in heaven's name had the lady made me come into town for that? Didn't she think she could tell it to me on the phone? And what was it about masturbation anyway? Was she seriously afraid of whatever stupidity the far right might try to make out of it?

Back at my office we took up the meeting where we had left off. But a few minutes into it another call came in, this time from Leon Panetta. Panetta didn't do any dances. "Dr. Elders," he said. "I don't believe we can stand any more of these remarks. They're just not acceptable. I want to have your resignation on my desk by two-thirty."

I think I was in a momentary state of shock. "Mr. Panetta," I said, "I'm not resigning unless my President asks me to."

"Well," he said, "the President's in Florida, and he's busy. I need your resignation this afternoon."

"I'm sorry," I said, "I'm not resigning until I talk to him."

I went back to the meeting, but they might have been able to read the disbelief on my face. It was obvious that Shalala wasn't just going to take it up with Panetta. Of course she had already had the discussion with him before she called me in. But I still wasn't thinking clearly about it—probably because of the triviality of what I had said and because I was so unprepared for the reaction. I was engaged in some truly controversial issues—I had been for a long time—but whether masturbation was part of human sexuality wasn't one of them.

Despite Panetta, I still wasn't thinking about resigning. I expected that Clinton and I would probably sit down and have a conversation. Of course the far right had been demanding my resignation practically every time they got on the air. But Clinton and I had stood side by side in some pretty rough fights. As far as I knew, there had never even been any rumors that he was considering asking me to leave. The single time anybody had said anything at all to me was after I had suggested studying legalization the previous December. Shalala had called me in then to express her disapproval, but that had been it.

So I wasn't really expecting Clinton to call. Even after the telephone began ringing with friends telling me they had just heard about my resignation on the radio and they wanted me to know they were sorry. I wondered whose office that news had leaked from. But I still couldn't really get myself to believe that the President was going to go along with it.

About an hour later, though, Clinton did call. "Joycelyn?"

"Yes, sir," I said.

"Joycelyn, I'm sorry this all is happening. But I hear there are all these remarks going on, and we can't have them. I want you to get your resignation into Panetta's office this afternoon."

"Mr. President? Do you know what I said?"

"Yes, they told me. I'm sorry, we've just got so many things, and I'm sorry."

And I said, "Well, thank you."

———

When I hung up, I called my secretary in and told her. "Don't say anything yet," I said. "Let me get myself glued together first." For the next half hour or so I didn't know what to think. I was even contemplating not resigning at all, and I got down the Commissioned Corps regulations to check the exact terms of the statutory appointment. Of course that passed quickly. My feelings of anger and disappointment took longer. This wasn't a job I had looked for. I had been asked to take it, and I had left a job I was happy with to do it. And Oliver had left a job he was happy with, to come up here to Washington, which was a place we didn't know.

Of course nobody had twisted my arm to come either, and I wasn't such a neophyte not to know what can happen in politics.

So the fact was that despite the hurt, I had no complaints coming. But at least, I thought, I would have handled this situation differently from the way the President did.

With time, though, I've come to feel more comfortable. Bill Clinton had nurtured my career and protected me for many years. But he had been torn up in the midterm elections, and in early December he probably still felt like the dogs were biting him. The Democrats had been swept out, and the Republicans were in. From what he could see, the American people, those who had voted, did not want to go the way he wanted to go. And he knew for sure that I was not going to change.

I still don't think that the President himself would have wanted me to leave. If it had just been him, nothing would have come of it. But as Donna Shalala liked to say, I was never her choice, and once the President's chief of staff decided I was a liability, it was just a matter of finding the opportunity.

———

It took me a little while to get back on my feet, but I've never been a person who looks back, and I had to make up my mind where I was going to land. This was over and done. The old preachers used to have a saying about tribulation. A bend in the road, they said, is not the end of the road. As Oliver and I gathered ourselves together to go back to Little Rock, I never had any doubt about that at all. The President has not been in touch with me since then, nor I with him. Honestly, I don't know what we would say to each other. I feel we both probably understand what happened.

Epilogue

After I resigned, one interviewer asked me whether I had any regrets. I don't. I left feeling that I gave the best I could give. I always tried to say what I believed to be the truth, without regard to whether it might be tactful or diplomatic. When I was surgeon general, I felt I had nothing to lose. I have even less to lose now that I am out of public service and back as a pediatric endocrinologist at the University of Arkansas. None of the essentials has changed. I'm a physician. I'm black and female. I've been poor. I've been through it. I'm still here, and I'm still in the fight.

The same interviewer asked if I felt I was on a mission. The answer is that I feel absolutely committed to the issues I have always been about: comprehensive health education, prevention of teenage pregnancy, early-childhood education, school-based clinics to make health care available for all children, a preventive approach to health care for everyone. These were my issues when I was director of public health in Arkansas and when I was surgeon general. They still are as I try to combine my life at the medical school with what sometimes seems like nonstop speaking engagements around the country. For me these aren't things of the moment; I've never been a politician. They are still my issues.

A great deal has happened since I left office. With House and Senate Republicans in the majority, the threat to the principles I have fought for has grown. Comprehensive health education has been opposed at every turn. The Republican budget targeted early-childhood education and cut Head Start. Research on AIDS and money for AIDS education and prevention have suffered. The AIDS epidemic is gathering speed, especially among blacks, women, and adolescents, but little is said about it. Out-of-wedlock teenage pregnancy, the key factor in the cycle of poverty, ignorance, and crime, is rising among our youngest girls, ages twelve to seventeen. Teenage pregnancy may be the single greatest threat to America's social fabric. But the government cannot effectively educate young people about sex and contraception because the religious right has entrenched itself in the Republican party and the religious right can't tolerate the idea.

Naturally I would prefer that every young person waited to become sexually active. But that's not realistic in today's world. The reality is that 54 percent of high school students engage in sexual intercourse. Do we write them off as lost causes not worth saving? Do we stand idly by while a million teenage girls become pregnant each year and five hundred thousand end their pregnancies by abortion? Do we ignore the growing incidence of STDs among young people and the tragedy of AIDS? I don't think so. That's not my kind of morality.

Personally I can't reconcile morality with doing nothing to stop the suffering around us. I don't believe that God intends us to let the ideal blind us to the real. I don't believe it's ethical simply to tell teenagers to say no and then write off the ones who don't. This is especially so since we know that often it's not the ones with active sexual lives who get into trouble; they tend to know how to take care of themselves. It's youngsters who try to experiment before they should, or make mistakes with alcohol, or are taken advantage of by someone older— young people whom we never adequately taught to protect themselves.

I don't think I'm expected to neglect a child because I disapprove of his or her behavior. Many young people are at risk because they are engaging in premature, unprotected sexual activity. I believe it is my responsibility as a Christian to set aside my personal judgment about when sex should begin, in order to promote programs and policies that protect the health of all children. I sometimes thought we should have just given the condom issue over to the Defense Department. They buy weapons all the time, not to start wars, but to defend the nation. I didn't give out condoms to precipitate sex, but to protect the country's most valuable resource, our young people, from AIDS, STDs, and unwanted pregnancy.

One of my points of contention with the religious right is that they are massively engaged on the abortion issue, yet you never see them out there fighting to provide adequate housing or to fund early-childhood education or to improve medical coverage for poor families. In my view, that does not show a will to protect our society's helpless and hopeless. On the contrary. To me that is not true but false morality. I challenge the Christian Coalition to put its resources into finding ways to care for children in need. If it did that, it would at least have the standing to argue about abortion. There are those in the antiabortion movement whose stand is part of a philosophy that includes opposition to the death penalty and a commitment to the poor. Those groups deserve respect, no matter how deeply I disagree with them about a woman's right to choose. But there are others whose moralizing is hollow because it is not accompanied by charity of the heart.

Those are the Ralph Reeds and Pat Buchanans and Jerry Falwells. They have nothing to do with values as I understand them and especially nothing to do with family values or Christian family values. Family values, to me, mean caring about others. Family values mean nurturing our nuclear and extended families. Everybody's family doesn't have to look like mine. We can have single-parent families. We can have same-sex families. But we must have families that support each other, take care of each other, protect each other, and respect each other. And we have to have public programs and policies that help them do that.

Because sooner or later a nation that does not take care of its youngest, eldest, and weakest will truly self-destruct.

The other reason the religious right disturbs me so badly is that its vision of its own rightness is an exclusive vision. In the 1992 Republican convention Pat Buchanan stood up and said that "there is a religious war going on in this country." In this war, he said, there is "the other side" and "our side." As much as some Republicans would like it not to be, the agenda of the social conservatives appeals to all those old-time prejudices against women, blacks, Jews, homosexuals, and immigrants. America, Buchanan said, is still "God's country." But we know who the people are that Pat Buchanan would welcome into his version of "God's country," and we know who they aren't. I'm not on that list. You may not be either.

Buchanan's speech back then put the country on notice. The country is still on notice. Now we have to decide if we want to regain control and keep America inclusive—with room for us all. Or do we want to turn it over to these self-righteous, self-appointed folk who have so little room for anybody different?

I feel so strongly about this because I've had an inside look at exclusion and inclusion both. I've been one, and I've been the other. Over the years I was always more drawn to action than to introspection. But now that I'm looking back, two things seem to stand out in my life. One is the help I've had from others. At every step I've had my Edith Irby Joneses and Ed Hugheses and Tom Butlers and my United Methodist women. And all these years I've had my husband, Oliver, to be my rock and my support. The second is that I, a child who might never have gotten off the cotton field, have been included in the American dream.

It's strange in a way to reflect on that. I see so much of the traditional portrait of America in the things that I have known in my life. The farm and the little country church, a loving mother and father who spent every ounce of their strength to feed their family and who watched their children rise from poverty to college and good jobs. All that could have come straight out of Norman Rockwell. Except that my American dream was in color.

I was among the first generation of African Americans who could even think about saying "my American dream." And even for me that was more a matter of luck than anything else. Once I got to medical school, I made it the way young white men traditionally did, by having a mentor who took a real interest in me and did what needed to be done to promote my career. But it was just my good fortune that I came along at the particular moment I did.

If I had come up ten years earlier, I never would have been picked to be chief pediatric resident at the University of Arkansas, or any resident. Chances are I never would have gotten into medical school at all. Ten years earlier black students in the South could go only to black medical schools. With just two, Meharry and Howard, it was almost impossible to get admitted. And if you did get in, there was almost no way to go from there into academic medicine. Those schools provided excellent clinical training, but they didn't have the resources to do much high-level medical research. The world of medical science would have been closed to me. I might have set up a practice in a black community or inner city and been a good doctor. But I never would have had the opportunities I had, never would have done the science and medicine I did, never would have had the life I've led.

But I came along at a time when some universities were beginning to take black students, even trying to recruit. With almost no black faculty members, medical schools were just starting to look for young African Americans to go into academic medicine. And I had the right bag of tricks for that moment: a feel for science, an ability to get along with people, and a determination not to fail. There was no affirmative action then, but a broad cultural change was under way. Fortunately for me I was there at the right time.

Some years later that social momentum got translated into the policy of affirmative action. Now twenty-five years have gone by, and there's a backlash. People want to get rid of affirmative action, nobody more than the social conservatives. Their main argument is that affirmative action should be scrapped because it supposedly favors unqualified blacks over qualified whites. We have a level playing field now, they argue, so why prolong such a racially divisive policy?

Well, I can tell you that most African Americans do not see affirmative action that way. We look at a history in this country of education and jobs going to white people simply because they were white, while untold numbers of talented black people were disregarded and swept aside. We see a playing field that for almost all this country's existence was not just slanted against blacks; they weren't even allowed on it so they could get into the game.

That's first. Secondly, the group affirmative action has helped most is not blacks but white women. I'm not saying that's bad. Far from it. Women have suffered their own long experience of exclusion from America's promises. When I served on the admissions committee at the medical school, I had to spend more time shouting to get women admitted than I did to get blacks in. But though women have been the chief beneficiaries of affirmative action, we never hear talk about how destructive the policy is to relations between the sexes, only to those between the races.

Most important, although nobody ever talks about it, the real significance of affirmative action is not that it advantages one group or another, but that it is medicine designed to cure America's ailing institutions. Historically the country's colleges, professional schools, businesses, and unions have been sick. They discriminated against minorities and women in favor of white men. In their prejudice they deprived themselves of the full available pool of talent, which hurt them, those they excluded, and the country they were meant to be serving.

Because their discrimination was embedded for so long, these institutions have needed help in healing themselves. The civil rights movement created a climate that allowed some of society's second-class citizens to go where they had previously been kept out. A few in my generation were able to swim the river. But the institutions themselves remained flawed at the center, despite their attempts to do better. Given that they were founded by white males to benefit white males and that their culture has always been a white male culture, how could it be different?

Changing institutions is a long-term business. Four hundred years of affirmative action in favor of white males have not been successfully countered by a twenty-five-year attempt to make sure minorities and women are included. That's why affirmative action is still needed. Habits die hard, even where the spirit is willing to change. Equality and fairness don't happen in the blinking of an eye. They take root slowly.

Maybe some people think we're there already. I don't. Look at the upper levels of management today, and you'll see that blacks and women barely exist. The same with upper-level faculty at today's law, business, and medical schools. Someone the other day showed me a photograph from the Boston *Globe,* the most liberal state's most liberal newspaper, a picture of ten women CEOs. If fairness had already dug itself deep into our institutions, we would never see such a picture. If equality were the norm, we'd never hear about this black professor or that black banker. They'd be too common to notice.

When affirmative action has done its job, it will wither away. No one will have to kill it because it will die its own natural death. Voting rights laws are not needed where everyone has the right to vote. Affirmative action makes no sense where institutional prejudice does not exist. But if you think we are already there, just look around.

All this having been said, the truth is that affirmative action is a philosophy that goes deeper than race, deeper than gender, and beyond institutions. It goes right to the heart of our democratic life.

No matter how wide the doors have swung, if you can't read, you're not going through. Thirty years ago we saw that the doors were closed and had to be opened. Now we know that so many of our youngsters will never be prepared to step through. White and black, boys and girls, it makes no difference. Sixty-five percent of our poor and ignorant and underserved are white.

White and black, they grow up in places where so often there's nobody to read them a book, nobody to see they do their homework, nobody to make sure they're fed properly or clothed decently. We can't wait for these children to get old enough to look for a job or think about college before we apply affirmative action. By then it's too late, for them and for us.

That's why I argue everywhere I go that resources have to be focused on our children—on Head Start and early enrichment and after-school programs. I want to be saying to this country something more than just "Yes, I made it, so you can too." Because the fact is that I had plenty of help: a stable family, a working community, teachers who cared, and a church that mattered. But this kind of help is not out there for so many of today's young people growing up in broken homes and broken communities. In a country as rich as ours we all have an obligation to do everything we can to try to balance this out, so these children too can have a chance to cross the river and see what it's like on the other side.

That's how I see a lot of what I've tried to do. In my own way I've done what I could to keep them healthy, to get them through school, and to give them hope. That's what I wanted for all those children I saw in the delta and up in Arkansas's mountains, the ones who were in my care when I was health director and the ones who came into my care when I was surgeon general. If I could keep them well, keep them from having children while they were still children themselves, and give them some hope they could go to college, that's what I wanted. That was my idea of affirmative action. After they got past that, they could take care of themselves.

When it comes right down to it, I don't really think of myself as a model for young black women. If anything, I hope to be some kind of example for disadvantaged young people of all kinds, for the kids who don't have the usual models they should be growing up with. I want us—you and I—to think of all those kids as our children. That's what I really want. When you pare away all the excess and get down to the core, that's what I am about.

Index